W0230571

Embryology

Text and
PowerPoint Presentation

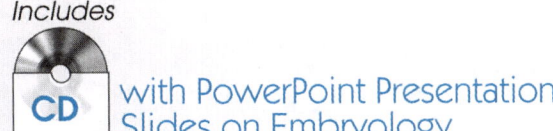

Includes

CD with PowerPoint Presentation
Slides on Embryology

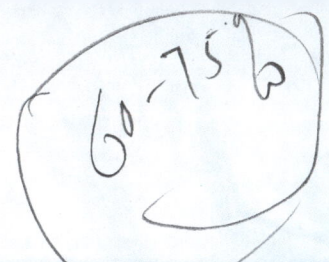

Embryology

Text and
PowerPoint Presentation

Chief Editor

S Saritha MBBS, MS (Anatomy)

Professor and Head
Department of Anatomy
Kamineni Academy of Medical Sciences and
Research Center, Hyderabad

Editor

TV Ramani MBBS, MD (Anatomy)

Assistant Professor
Department of Anatomy
Kamineni Academy of Medical Sciences and
Research Center, Hyderabad

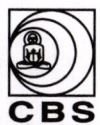

CBS

CBS Publishers & Distributors Pvt Ltd

New Delhi • Bengaluru • Chennai • Kochi • Kolkata • Mumbai
Hyderabad • Jharkhand • Nagpur • Patna • Pune • Uttarakhand

Disclaimer

Science and technology are constantly changing fields. New research and experience broaden the scope of information and knowledge. The editors have tried their best in giving information available to them while preparing the material for this book. Although all efforts have been made to ensure optimum accuracy of the material, yet it is quite possible some errors might have been left uncorrected. The publisher, the printer and the editors will not be held responsible for any inadvertent errors or inaccuracies.

Embryology
Text and
PowerPoint Presentation

ISBN: 978-93-87085-89-3

Copyright © Chief Editor and Publisher

First Edition: 2018

All rights reserved. No part of this book may be reproduced or transmitted in any form or by any means, electronic or mechanical, including photocopying, recording, or any information storage and retrieval system without permission, in writing, from the editors and the publisher.

Published by Satish Kumar Jain and produced by Varun Jain for

CBS Publishers & Distributors Pvt Ltd

4819/XI Prahlad Street, 24 Ansari Road, Daryaganj, New Delhi 110 002, India.
Ph: 23289259, 23266861, 23266867   Website: www.cbspd.com
Fax: 011-23243014   e-mail: delhi@cbspd.com; cbspubs@airtelmail.in.

Corporate Office: 204 FIE, Industrial Area, Patparganj, Delhi 110 092
Ph: 4934 4934   Fax: 4934 4935   e-mail: publishing@cbspd.com; publicity@cbspd.com

Branches

- **Bengaluru:** Seema House 2975, 17th Cross, K.R. Road, Banasankari 2nd Stage, Bengaluru 560 070, Karnataka
  Ph: +91-80-26771678/79   Fax: +91-80-26771680   e-mail: bangalore@cbspd.com
- **Chennai:** 7, Subbaraya Street, Shenoy Nagar, Chennai 600 030, Tamil Nadu
  Ph: +91-44-26680620, 26681266   e-mail: chennai@cbspd.com
- **Kochi:** Ashana House, No. 39/1904, AM Thomas Road, Valanjambalam, Ernakulam 682 016, Kochi, Kerala
  Ph: +91-484-4059061-65   Fax: +91-484-4059065   e-mail: kochi@cbspd.com
- **Kolkata:** 6/B, Ground Floor, Rameswar Shaw Road, Kolkata-700 014, West Bengal
  Ph: +91-33-22891126, 22891127, 22891128   e-mail: kolkata@cbspd.com
- **Mumbai:** 83-C, Dr E Moses Road, Worli, Mumbai-400018, Maharashtra
  Ph: +91-22-24902340/41   Fax: +91-22-24902342   e-mail: mumbai@cbspd.com

Representatives

- **Hyderabad** 0-9885175004
- **Jharkhand** 0-9811541605
- **Nagpur** 0-9021734563
- **Patna** 0-9334159340
- **Pune** 0-9623451994
- **Uttarakhand** 0-9716462459

Printed at: Mudrak, Patparganj, Delhi, India

Preface

I am pleased to introduce this new concept publication *Embryology* in the form of PowerPoint slides accompanied by relevant text material on the topics described in the PPt slides. These slides are simplified with scientific material in human development.

I have made efforts to give rich, clear and precise orientation and interpretation in each section with animation, wherever possible, for understanding of the undergraduate and postgraduate medical students as well as the teaching faculty.

This endeavor would have been lost in the ocean but for her husband, Dr Kumarswamy, for his constant inspiration and endurance.

I express my deep sense of gratitude to my teachers for their blessings. I also express my deep love to my daughter Dr K Kshitija and her junior staff Dr TV Ramani for constant support in preparing the PowerPoint slides and the related text material.

I will regard as a reward if the PowerPoint presentation on human embryology receives constructive criticism for improvement.

S Saritha
Chief Editor

Contents

Section 3 Embryology of Cardiovascular System Derived from Mesoderm

General Embryology

1

Introduction to General Embryology

Human developmental process represents an integration of complex phenomena. The study of these phenomena is called *embryology*. It deals with prenatal stages of development starting from fertilization of ovum to birth of new individual. Fertilization from a single cell the zygote changes to a multicellular baby in the period of 9 months. New life begins as zygote in the uterine tube of female. Zygote is formed by union of sperm (male gamete) with ovum (female gamete) known as fertilization.

Gametes are haploid cells with 23 chromosomes (22 autosomes + 1 sex chromosome) present in nucleus. Where as spermatogonium or oogonium cells including all somatic cells are diploid cells with 46 chromosomes (23 pairs, i.e. 22 pairs of autosomes and 1 pair of sex chromosomes). Gametes are formed in the gonads the ovary (in female) or testis (in males). Gametes are derived from stem cells in embryo primordial germ cells (PGCs).

It appears in the epiblast layer of embryo. PGCs appear in epiblast layer—1st week of IUL → 2nd week of IUL → endoderm of yolk sac → 4th week of IUL → they next migrate to the developing gonads by 5th week of IUL and settle down in the gonads. PMGs are diploid with 46 chromosomes. Divide by 2 phases of meiotic divisions or reduction division → form gametes (ovum or sperm) with haploid chromosomes (23). Conversion of primordial germ cells to gametes is known as **gametogenesis**.

Oogenesis is the process of formation of oocyte (ovum) from oogonia which is derived from PGCs within the ovary. Oogenesis begins in the ovaries of female fetus, i.e. before birth and it is completed at the time of puberty.

Spermatogenesis is the process of formation of sperm from spermatogonia which is derived from PGCs in the testis. Spermatogenesis begins in the testis at the time of puberty in males and it completed by 74 days.

Fertilization: Union of ovum and sperm takes place in the ampulla of uterine tube. Preparation for fertilization gametes (ovum or sperm):

1. Meiosis
2. Cytodifferentiation.
   - Restores the chromosomal no. 46
   - It determines sex of zygote at time of fertilization. Y bearing sperm fertilizes ovum, it results in male zygote and X bearing sperm fertilizes ovum, it results in female zygote.
   - Initiates cleavage of zygote
   - XX sex pair individual is genetically female.
   - XY sex pair individual is genetically male.
   - One from each pair derived from maternal gamete (oocyte), one from paternal gamete (sperm).

Each gamete has haploid (23) and union of gametes is fertilization which restores diploid (46).

CELL DIVISION

It involves two distinct events:

Division of nucleus: Karyokinesis and division of cytoplasm: Cytokinesis.

Nuclear division: It occurs in 2 ways:

I. *Direct division*: Amitotic division—nuclear material is distributed randomly to resultant daughter cells. It occurs only in pathological cells.

II. *Indirect division*

1. *Mitotic division (equation division)*: It occurs in all somatic cells and results in distribution of identical copies of parent cell's genome to two daughter cells.

2. *Meiosis or reduction division*: It occurs in formation of gametes (ovum and sperm) gametogenesis. Results in conversion of primary oocyte → ovum and primary spermatocyte → sperms. It results in distribution of half the number of chromosomes.

Cell cycle (20–24 hours) is the period of time between the birth of a cell. Cell that undergoes division regularly pass through interphase → mitosis → interphase → mitosis.

One complete passage through interphase and mitosis is termed as cell cycle. Cell cycle has 4 distant phases: G1, S, G2 and M.

G1, S and G2 are known as interphase. At the end of interphase → M phase occurs, giving two daughter cells.

Entire cell cycle takes 20–24 hours. Mitosis division (M phase) takes 1–2 hours.

Mitosis occurs in all somatic cells and PGCs. One cell divides into 2 daughter cells that are genetically identical to parent cell.

Mitosis has 4 stages: Prophase, metaphase, anaphase and telophase.

Significance of Mitosis

1. Genetic stability ensures continuous succession of identical cells through generations.
2. Growth and development of the body.
3. Regeneration, replacement repair helps in regeneration of new cells to replace the dead cells.

Meiosis or Reduction Division: Maturation of Sex Cells

Meiosis is a special type of cell division that takes place only in reproductive organs to produce gametes → haploid number of chromosomes.

It involves two sequential divisions

Meiosis I: Heterotypical division. DNA—tetraploid in amount; chromosomes number is diploid.

Prophase I: Long and complex phase which differs from mitotic prophase. It is divided into 5 substages: Leptotene, zygotene, pachytene, diplotene and diakinesis. Followed by metaphase I, anaphase I and telophase. At the end of meiosis I each daughter cell contains 23 double-stranded chromosomes. Two haploid cells and diploid amount of DNA.

Meiosis II: Homotypical division just like mitotic except no DNA replication. At the end of meiosis II, there are four daughter cells, each with a haploid set of chromosomes and haploid amount of DNA. Each daughter cell is genetically distinct from the others and from the parent cell.

Oogenesis: In human meiosis I, primary oocyte remains in diplotene stage: 5 months of IUL.

Remain in this stage till the period prior to ovulation. Some for decades even up to 50 years. Meiosis II is completed only at the time of fertilization.

APPLIED OF MEIOTIC DIVISION

Genetic variation in population: Exchange of genes between homologous chromosomes redistributes genetic material. Random distribution of homologous chromosomes to daughter cells. To provide each gamete with haploid number of chromosomes and half the amount of DNA.

- *Sexual reproduction:* Because of meiosis chromosomal number is maintained in species.
- *Hybrid vigor:* It helps to maintain vigor in progeny through sexual reproduction.

2

Gametogenesis: Oogenesis

Oogenesis is the process of formation of oocyte (ovum) from oogonia which is derived from PGCs within the ovary.

Spermatogenesis is the process of formation of sperm from spermatogonia which is derived from PGCs in the testis.

PGCs (TDF) with Y chromosome reach undifferentiated gonad, the gonad differentiates to testes and absence of Y gonads form ovaries. Primordial germ cells are pluripotent cells, fail to reach gonadal ridge leads to gonadal dysgenesis.

In preparation for fertilization germ cells undergo: Gametogenesis: Meiotic I and meiotic II.

The Reduction Division

1. Oogenesis or spermatogenesis.
2. Cytodifferentiation.

The formation, development and maturation of an ovum is oogenesis. Maturation of oocytes begins before birth, accelerates at puberty and ends at menopause.

Meiotic I starts in primary oocyte in IUL → 5 months and completed just before ovulation.

Meiotic II of secondary oocyte is completed just before fertilization.

As a result of two meiotic divisions: One primary oocyte gives rise to 4 daughter cells, each with 22 + X chromosome.

Oogenesis is a process whereby oogonia differentiate into mature oocyte.

1. **Prenatal maturation** begins before birth
2. **Postnatal maturation** continues at puberty.

Only one of these develops into mature gamete ovum and others form 3 polar bodies without cytoplasm (disintegrates during subsequent development and their biological inert).

PGCs (endoderm) reach ovary (5th week of IUL in female embryo), differentiate into oogonia.

Oogonia undergo number of mitotic divisions. End of 3rd month of IUL all oogonia arranged in clusters surrounded by layer of flat epithelial follicular cells originate surface epithelium of ovary (mesoderm). All oogonia in one cluster are derived → single PGC.

5th month of IUL total number of germ cells in the ovary, 7 million. Majority of oogonia and primary oocyte degenerate. 7th month of IUL all surviving primary oocyte → enter prophase I of meiotic division and arrested at diplotene stage.

Total number of primordial follicle with primary oocyte in diplotene—at birth is 600,000–800,000 (6–8 L).

During childhood, most of oocytes become atretic and only 40,000 are present at beginning of puberty.

Only 500 will be ovulated during entire reproductive life of an female individual (15–45th years).

At puberty (11–15 years), 15–20 primordial follicles begin to mature and pass through 3 stages:

1. Primary or preantral follicle.
2. Secondary or antral follicle.
3. Graafian or preovulatory follicle.

Graafian follicle is formed and luteinizing hormone (LH) from anterior pituitary → induces primary oocyte completes 1st meiotic division results in formation of 2 daughter cells of unequal size each with double-stranded 23 chromosomes.

One cell is secondary oocyte receives most of cytoplasm and other cell is 1st polar body receives practically none.

Secondary oocyte enters 2nd meiotic division without DNA replication. 2nd meiotic arrests in metaphase approximately 3 hours before ovulation.

Shedding of secondary oocyte in 2nd meiotic division surrounded ZP and corona radiata marks the ovulation (14th day of menstrual cycle).

Meiotic II is completed only if secondary oocyte is fertilized (ampulla of uterine tube), otherwise the cell degenerates approximately 24 hours after ovulation.

1st polar body may or may not undergo 2nd meiotic division, but it is seen that fertilized ovum is accompanied by 3rd polar bodies.

SPERMATOGENESIS

Maturation of male gametes in the wall of seminiferous tubules. Starts at puberty (14–18th years). Process of formation of spermatozoa from the PGCs → gives rise to stem cell spermatogonia → presents in the wall of seminiferous tubules of testes. PGCs remain dormant in the seminiferous tubules till puberty.

1. PGSc
2. Spermatogonia divide mitotically
3. Primary spermatocytes (46) which enter 1st meiotic and give rise to two equal haploid cells.
4. Secondary spermatocyte with 23 (22 + X and 22 + Y). Secondary spermatocytes immediately followed by 2nd meiotic division giving rise → spermatids (2 with X and 2 with Y).

Spermatids change into highly motile sperms by spermatogenesis forming → sperms head (nucleus), neck, middle piece and tail.

Spermatogenesis consists of three stages

1. Spermatocytosis (16 days): PGCs → spermatogonia → primary spermatocyte.
2. Meiosis I (24 days) and II (few hours). Primary spermatocyte → secondary spermatocyte → spermatids.
3. Spermiogenesis (30–34 days). Spermatids → spermatozoa.

The time required for spermatogonium to become a mature spermatozoon is approximately 74 days.

Approximately 300 million sperm cells are produced daily. Fully formed spermatozoa enter the lumen of seminiferous tubules, from here pushed towards the epididymis by contractions of seminiferous tubules → vas deferens → ejaculatory duct → emitted via male urethra.

Maternal contributions to the fertilized oocyte (zygote)

- Half of zygotic genome
- Maternal mitochondria
- Maternal nucleolus
- Maternal ribosome

Paternal contributions to the fertilized oocyte (zygote)

- Half of zygotic genome
- Centrioles

Fertilization

FIRST WEEK OF DEVELOPMENT: OVULATION TO IMPLANTATION

Gestation period subdivided into 3 stages

1. Germinal period: Extends first 3 weeks of development
2. Embryonic period: Extends from 4 to 8th weeks.
3. Fetal period: 3rd month up to termination of pregnancy.

1. **Germinal period:** Extends first 3 weeks of development. It begins with fertilization and it includes:
   a. Cleavage → morula, blastocyst and implantation (1st week).
   b. Bilaminar disc—2nd week and trilaminar disc—3rd week
   c. Differentiation of trophoblast and chorion.
2. **Embryonic period:** Extends from 4 to 8th weeks → crucial period. It is characterized by changes in shape and external appearance. Three germ layers undergo individual differentiation and most of tissues and organs of the body are formed.
3. **Fetal period:** 3rd month up to termination of pregnancy. There is rapid growth of fetus.

INTRODUCTION

Fertilization is a process by which male gamete spermatozoon and female gamete ovum (the pronuclei) fuse to form zygote. It occurs at ampullary end of uterine tube.

Spermatozoa are not able to fertilize the oocyte immediately upon arrival in FGT but undergoes.
1. Capacitation
2. Acrosome reaction.

Three barriers protect the female gamete

- **Corona radiata**
- **Zona pellucida**
- **Vitelline membrane (plasma membrane)**

  Sperm has to pass 3 barriers to fertilize.

Phases of fertilization include

1. *Penetration of corona radiata*: Only a capacitated sperm passes freely through corona radiata, binds to zona pellucida (ZP).
2. *Penetration of zona pellucida*: Zona pellucida is glycoprotein shell surrounding the egg, that induces the acrosome reaction.
3. *Fusion of oocyte and sperm cell membranes*: As soon as sperm and oocyte plasma membranes come in contact and fuse. Secondary oocyte completes its 2nd meiotic division.

About 200–300 million spermatozoa deposited in the FGT. Only 300–500 (1%) reach the site of fertilization (2–7 hours). Only one sperm is needed for fertilization and others aid in fertilizing sperm in penetrating the barriers protecting the female gamete.

Spermatozoa rapidly pass → vagina → uterus → ampullary end of uterine tube, by muscular contractions of uterus and UT and also by their own propulsion (2–7 hours).

Completion of 2nd meiotic division of secondary oocyte, results → mature ovum with 2nd polar body (extruded). Nucleus of mature ovum → female pronucleus containing haploid number of chromosomes 22 + X. Spermatozoon moves forwards close to female pronucleus. It becomes swollen and forms male pronucleus (22 + X or Y) tail detaches and degenerates. Results in fertilization → zygote.

Morphologically male and female pronuclei are indistinguishable, replicate DNA lose their nuclear membrane and eventually come in close contact. Zygote enter into 1st meiotic division → two cells stage of zygote is the 1st meiotic division and it initiation of cleavage.

Main Results of Fertilization: Five Factors

1. Completion of 2nd meiotic division of secondary oocyte.
2. Restoration of diploid number of chromosomes.
3. Determination of sex of new individual
4. Initiation of cleavage: Division of zygote occurs mitotically, forming morula.
5. Determination of polarity of the embryo in line of entry of spermatozoon probably decides cephalocaudal polarity of the zygote.

Cleavage

- Once the zygote reached two cells stage, it undergoes a series of mitotic division resulting increasing the number of cells known as morula.
- Two cells derived from first cleavage of zygote are of unequal size.
- Large cell divides first, than small cell, forming four cells stage.
- Inner cells of morula give rise to embryo proper. Surrounding outer cell mass forms the trophoblast which later forms placenta. Morula 16 cells stage on the 4th day (96 hours) enters the uterine cavity. Morula enveloped by ZP. Fluid begins to penetrate through the ZP into intercellular spaces of inner cell mass.
- These spaces coalesce to form a single cavity of the blastocele.
- Embryo is also known as blastocyst (70–100 cells).

Blastocyst (5th Day)

Inner cell mass is referred to as embryoblast.

Outer cell mass is referred to as trophoblast which is flat epithelial surrounding the inner cell mass, forms wall of blastocyst. Trophoblast cells over embryonic pole begin to penetrate cells of uterine mucosa on the 6–7th day of fertilization.

Out of 107 cells

- 8 cells form embryoblast.
- 30 cells form polar trophoblast
- Rest 69 cells persist as mural trophoblast.

Implantation (6–7th Day)

Polar trophoblast (embryonic pole) begins to penetrate uterine mucosa (decidua) about 6–7th day. Uterus at the time of implantation is in secretory phase. Blastocyst implants between junction fundus and posterior wall of body of uterus. If fertilization fails to occur, menstrual phase occurs.

End of the first week of development the human zygote passes through the morula and blastocyst stages and begins implantation in the uterine mucosa.

Clinical Correlation

Barrier techniques prevent pregnancy

- Male condom: Made up of latex containing chemical spermicides.
- Female condom: Made up of polyurethane which lines vagina, others diaphragm, cervical cap, etc.
- Contraceptive pill (female): A combination of estrogen and progesterone which inhibits ovulation.
- Male pill contains androgen which prevents FSH and LH secretion and stops sperm production.
- Intrauterine device (IUD) placed in uterine cavity prevents pregnancy.
- Vasectomy and tubectomy.

4

Bilaminar Germ Disc

2nd week of development (8–14th days)

1st week of development: Fertilization occurs 24 hours after ovulation. Implantation of blastocyst occurs on 6–7 days after fertilization. However, embryo of same fertilization age does not develop at same rate. Implantation provides nutrition to growing embryo from maternal blood. Initially nutrition of the embryo is by diffusion and later through the development of placenta.

During 2nd week the trophoblast and embryoblast of blastocyst differentiate individually although one is dependent on other for development. Blastocyst is gradually embedded in endometrial stroma (decidua) by the histolytic action of trophoblast. At the embryonic pole of blastocyst grows deep in endometrial stroma.

Blastocyst (2nd week): Changes in trophoblast and embryoblast

- 8th day of development
- 9–10th day is lacunar stage
- 11–12th day → uteroplacental circulation
- 13–14th day → villous system

8th day of development

1. Blastocyst is partially embedded
2. Trophoblast differentiates into two layers: Cytotrophoblast and syncytiotrophoblast.

3. Embryoblast also differentiates into 2 layers: Hypoblast layer and epiblast layer, i.e. formation of bilaminar disc.
4. Amniotic cavity.

9–10th Day is Lacunar Stage

1. Blastocyst is more deeply embedded by fibrium coagulum.
2. Trophoblast: Embryonic pole: Vacuoles appear in syncytium, fuse and form large lacunae.
3. Embryoblast: Abembryonic pole: Heuser's membrane, primitive yolk sac.

11–12th Day → Uteroplacental Circulation

1. Blastocyst is completely embedded.
2. Trophoblast: Syncytiotrophoblast cells penetrate deeper into endometrium and erode the endothelial lining of maternal capillaries. Maternal blood begins to flow establishing uteroplacental circulation.
3. Embryoblast: Primary yolk sac outer side → extraembryonic mesoderm → extraembryonic coelomic cavity.

13–14th Day → Villous System

1. Trophoblast: Primary villi and lacunae are known as intervillous spaces.
2. Embryoblast: Hypoblast cells next produce additional cells → new cavity known as definitive yolk sac or secondary yolk sac.
3. Expansion of chorionic cavity.

Clinical Correlation

Syncytiotrophoblast is responsible for production of hormones, i.e. human chorionic gonadotropin (hCG). 2nd week hCG is sufficient to be detected in urine and radioimmunoassay which serves as basis for pregnancy testing.

Trilaminar Germ Disc

THIRD WEEK OF DEVELOPMENT: 15TH TO 21ST DAYS

Most significant changes in the 3rd week of gestation is conversion of bilaminar disc to trilaminar disc.

Gastrulation where in the embryo establishes 3 germ layers; the ectoderm, mesoderm and endoderm. The changes also occur in trophoblast, i.e. primary villi → secondary villi → tertiary villi. The gastrulation begins with the formation of primitive streak (16th day) in the midline at the caudal end, on the surface of epiblast cells.

Epiblast Layer (Primitive Ectoderm)

Cells differentiate into 3 functional zones:

1. Cells of cephalic zone and peripheral margin of disc form a semilunar area → forms the surface ectoderm.
2. Within concavity of surface ectoderm → neuroectodermal cells → entire structure → gives rise to CNS.
3. Pluripotent cells → caudal region.

Primitive streak is formed by active migration and invagination of pluripotent epiblast cells.

Primitive streak acts primary organizer and induces the differentiation of

1. Notochord
2. Intraembryonic mesoderm.

Some cells from primitive streak displace hypoblast cells thereby forming embryonic endoderm → 3rd germ layer.

Some cells lie between ectoderm and endoderm and form intraembryonic mesoderm → 2nd germ layer → or secondary mesoderm.

Surface ectoderm forms the epidermis of skin and neuro-ectoderm → forms CNS.

Together form definitive ectoderm germ layer → 1st germ layer.

Thus, epiblast layer through the process of gastrulation is source of 3 germ layers in the embryo

1. Ectoderm
2. Mesoderm
3. Endoderm

Cells of these germ layers → ectoderm, mesoderm and endoderm give rise to all tissues and organs of embryo.

Prochordal plates (14th day) are columnar cells derived from first cells that migrate through primitive node in midline and move in cephalic direction. Prochordal plate will later important for induction of forebrain. It establishes craniocaudal axis of embryo (central axis) and bilateral symmetry of the embryo. It forms the buccopharyngeal membrane—14th day.

Formation of notochord (16th–22nd days)

Notochord is the forerunner of midline axis.

1. Important in bilateral symmetry.
2. Inducer and differentiation of neural tube formation.
3. Acts in development of primitive vertebral column.

The process by which the hollow notochordal process is transformed into a solid notochord between 16th and 22nd days.

Definitive notochord (midline) extends from prechordal plate and caudally to primitive node.

Remnants of Notochord

In adult persists:

- Nucleus pulposus in intervertebral disc and apical ligament of dens of axis.
- Chordoma: Tumors arising from remnants of notochord, formed cranial or caudal.
- Cloacal membrane—16th day: Formed at the caudal end of embryonic disc.
- This membrane is similar to the buccopharyngeal membrane.

Changes in the Trophoblast during 3rd Week

1. Beginning of 3rd week trophoblast is characterized by primary villi (consisting of cytotrophoblast core covered by syncytium layer of cells).
2. EE mesoderm cells penetrate the core of primary villi and grow in the direction of decidua → villi are secondary.
3. By end of 3rd week mesodermal cells in core of villi differentiate into blood vessels and blood cells, forming villous capillary system → tertiary villi.

Tertiary villi are the definitive villi and always vascular and villous capillary system.

Capillaries in tertiary villi make contact with capillaries developing in mesoderm of chorionic plate and with the connecting stalk. Vessels of connecting stalk establish connection with intraembryonic circulating system which is also simultaneously developing → placenta villi connecting with the embryo.

Heart Begins to Beat at the Beginning of 4th Week of Development

Establishment of body axes: Anteroposterior or dorsoventral and left–right body axes take place during the period of gastrulation. Primitive streak and primitive node regulate the genes.

Clinical Correlation

Teratogenesis associated with gastrulation. 3rd week, primitive streak is highly sensitive stage for teratogenic insult. Fate maps for various organs are established during 3rd week of development.

Embryonic Period

Period of organogenesis: 4 to 8th weeks of development

It is the time when each of 3 germ layers, i.e. ectoderm, mesoderm and endoderm gives rise to number of specific tissues and organs.

End of embryonic period; main organs and embryonic folds are formed as a result embryo changes in its major features. The external body of embryo is recognized by the end of 2nd month (8th week.)

Age of Embryo

1. Presomite period → 15 to 20th days (3rd week)
2. Somite period: 20 to 30th days (4–5th week)
3. Postsomite period → expressed as:
     i. Crown rump length (CRL) → sitting height.
     ii. Crown heel length (CHL) → standing height.

Presomite period 15 to 20th days is related to development of

1. Primitive streak
2. Notochord
3. Intraembryonic mesoderm.

Somite period 20–30th days (4 to 5th week)

- 42 to 44 pairs of somites appear.
- Derived from intraembryonic mesoderm.
- Either side of notochord.

DERIVATIVES OF ECTODERM (ONE GERM LAYER) AT BEGINNING OF 3RD WEEK

Surface Ectoderm and Neuroectoderm

Prechordal cells induce the overlying neuroectoderm to thicken to form neural plate.

Neurulation is process whereby the neural plate forms neural tube.

The stages of neurulation include the formation of

Neural plate, neural groove, neural folds and fusion, neural crest cells and neural tube.

Neurulation begins during the late 3rd week (20th day), ends by the end of 4th week (28th day). It is mainly induced by the notochord.

1. Neural plate first appears: Cranial to the primitive node.
2. Lateral edges of neural plate become elevated to form neural folds and depression mid-region forms the neural groove.
3. Tips of neural groove are lined by specialized cells. Neural crest cells, which are continuous with surface ectoderm. Neural groove extends from Hensen's node to buccopharyngeal membrane.
4. Development proceeds neural folds approach each other in midline where they fuse → neural tube.
5. Fusion begins at cervical region or neck region (5th somite) and proceeds cranially and caudally, as a result neural tube is formed.
6. Cephalic and caudal ends communicate with amniotic cavity by the way anterior and posterior neuropores. Neuropores provide nutrition to neural tube as blood vascular system is yet to develop.
7. Closure of cranial or anterior neuropore occurs at 25th day (20 somite stage).

Closure of caudal or posterior neuropore occurs at 28th day (25 somite stage)

The cranial one-third of the neural tube represents the future brain. The caudal two-thirds represent the future spinal cord.

Neural crest cells: As neural folds elevate and fuse, cells at lateral border of neuroectoderm begin dissociate and form neural crest cell population.
1. Craniofacial skeleton
2. Neurons for cranial ganglia (sensory ganglia)
3. Glial cells
4. Connective tissue of head and neck
5. Conotruncal cushions of heart.

   Neural crest cells are fundamentally important and contribute to so many organs and tissues and considered as 4th germ layer.

Surface Ectoderm Placodes

By time neural tube is closed two bilateral ectodermal thickenings. Otic and lens placodes are seen at cephalic region of embryo.

   Otic placodes develop into membranous labyrinth of internal ear hearing and equilibrium (vestibular apparatus).

   Lens placodes: During 5th week and forms lens of eyeball.

   Surface ectoderm forms the epidermis of skin.

Clinical Correlation

Neural tube defects (NTDs): These result when neural tube closure fails to occur.
1. Cranial region: Anencephaly → most of brain fails to form.
2. Caudal in cervical region onwards: Spina bifida → most common in lumbosacral region.

Summary of Ectoderm Derivatives

1. CNS and PNS including cranial, spinal and ANS ganglia.
2. Sensory epithelium of ear, nose and eye.

3. Epidermis, hair, nails, sebaceous and sweat glands.
4. Epithelial lining of cheek, gums, enamel of teeth, roof of mouth, nasal cavity, paranasal sinuses, salivary glands (parotid), terminal part of anal canal and urethra.
5. Pituitary gland and mammary gland.
6. External acoustic meatus, outer layer of tympanic membrane and membranous labyrinth of internal ear.
7. Corneal epithelium, conjunctiva, lacrimal gland, nasolacrimal duct, lens and retina.
8. Muscles of iris and arrector pilorum.

DERIVATIVES OF MESODERMAL GERM LAYER

Intraembryonic mesoderm (secondary mesoderm) is derived from caudal part of primitive streak—16th day. Detachment of cells from the primitive streak forms mesodermal cells between ectoderm and endoderm. Intraembryonic mesoderm layer forms a thin sheet of loosely woven tissue on each side of midline or notochord.

It is subdivided by longitudinal groove into 3 parts by 17th day

1. Paraxial mesoderm (medial)
2. Intermediate mesoderm (middle)
3. Lateral plate mesoderm (lateral)

Paraxial mesoderm—3rd week; begins to organize into segments

It forms bilateral solid cord of cells extending along side of notochord and beneath neural tube. Later begins to organize into segments. First pair of somite appear in cephalic region (occipital region—20th day) of embryo and proceeds cephalocaudal direction. Somites appear between 20–30th days of development. From here onwards, somites appear craniocaudal sequence. At the rate of 3 pairs/day until end → 30th day or 5th week 42–44 pairs are present.

Cranialmost 3–4 somite pairs are occipital. Somites situated by the side of hindbrain.

It helps in formation of skull base.

Somites are in pairs → 42 to 44 pairs

- Occipital → 4
- Cervical → 8
- Thoracic → 12
- Lumbar → 5
- Sacral → 5
- Coccygeal → 8–10
- 1st occipital and last 5–7 coccygeal somites disappear.

Remaining somites (35–37) form the axial skeleton

Each somite forms:

1. Its own sclerotome (cartilage and bone component)
2. Its own myotome (segmental muscle component)
3. Dermatome (forms the dermis of skin)
4. It has own segmental spinal nerve.

Intermediate Mesoderm

Temporarily connects paraxial mesoderm and lateral plate mesoderm. It forms urogenital structures; gives rise to urinary system and gonads.

Lateral Plate Mesoderm

Splits into parietal (somatic) and visceral (splanchnic) layers which line intraembryonic cavity. It forms pericardial, pleural and peritoneal cavities.

Intraembryonic Blood Vessels and Blood Cells

These are derived from mesoderm by 3rd of development surrounding yolk sac.

Blood circulation in embryo and heart starts beating—21st or 22nd day.

Mesoderm forms both epithelia and mesenchyme.

Intraembryonic Mesoderm Derivatives

- All connective tissues including skeletal system.
- Teeth exception enamel (ectoderm).
- All muscles of the body except muscles of iris and arrector pilorum.
- Cardiovascular system (CVS) and lymphatic system.
- Urogenital system except most urinary bladder, prostate and urethra.
- Cortex of suprarenal.
- Gonads (except primordial germ cells)
- Mesothelium lining of peritoneal, pleural and pericardial cavities.

ENDODERMAL GERM CELL LAYER DERIVATIVES

The folding of embryo is a significant event of primitive form of human body. Starts end of 3rd → end of 4th week. As a result cephalocaudal foldings and lateral foldings flat embryonic disc which becomes cylindrical embryo.

Gastrointestinal tract is main organ derived from endodermal germ layer. Endoderm covers the ventral surface of the embryo and roofs of the yolk sac.

Folding of embryo occurs in the 4th week of IUL

1. Rapid growth of brain vesicles, flat trilaminar embryonic disc begins to fold cephalocaudal direction, thus establishing the head and tail folds.
2. Disc also folds in transverse direction due to development of somites → lateral folds. Folds occur end of 3rd week of development.
3. As a result of cephalocaudal folds, large portions of endodermal germ layer and yolk sac are incorporated into body of embryo to form gut tube.
4. Part of yolk sac within the embryonic folds forms primitive gut. The gut closed cranially by oropharyngeal membrane and caudally by cloacal membrane.

Primitive gut tube is divided into 3 regions → foregut within head fold and hindgut within tail fold. Midgut communicates with yolk sac by vitelline intestinal duct.

Stomadeum (ectoderm): Surface depression separated from pharynx (endoderm) by BP membrane.

Proctodeum (ectoderm): Surface depression separated from upper part of anal canal (endoderm) by cloacal membrane. Yolk sac cavity is reduced in size and undergoes hour-glass constriction by convergence of folds on ventral surface of embryo.

Extraembryonic part of yolk sac forms umbilical vesical, which connected to primitive gut by vitellointestinal duct. Ventral body closes completely except for umbilical region. Initially there is wide communication is between embryo and yolk sac, later it becomes constricted into a long vitelline duct.

Cephalocaudal and lateral folding is the part of allantois (diverticulum), is also incorporated into the body of embryo, where it forms cloaca.

Derivatives of Foregut

1. Mucous membrane of tongue.
2. Epithelial lining of pharynx, esopharynx, stomach, duodenum up to ampulla of Vater.
3. Epithelial lining of respiratory system.
4. Auditory tube and tympanic cavity.
5. Parenchyma of tonsil, thyroid, parathyroid, thymus, liver and pancreas.

Derivatives of Midgut

1. Epithelial lining of duodenum distal to ampulla of Vater, rest of small intestine, caecum, appendix, ascending colon and right two-thirds of transverse colon.
2. Meckel's diverticulum (persists vitellointestinal duct).

Derivatives of Hindgut

1. Mucous membrane of transverse colon from left one-third to upper part of anal canal.
2. Mucous membrane of urinary bladder, urethra and parenchyma of prostate.
3. Epithelium of vagina.
4. Primitive sex cells derived from dorsal wall of hindgut.

Endodermal Derivatives

- Epithelial lining of GIT.
- Epithelial lining of respiratory system.
- Epithelial lining of urethra and urinary bladder.
- Prostate and vagina.
- Liver and pancreas.
- Thyroid and parathyroid glands.
- Primordial germ cells.

Clinical Correlation

The period of organogenesis (embryogenesis) is between 3rd to 8th weeks, which is critical period for normal development.

Stem cell populations are established for each organ of primordia.

These interactions are sensitive to insult from genetic and environmental in influences, leading to most gross structural birth defects → congenital abnormalities.

Fetal Period

This period begins from 9th week or 3rd month to birth. Fetal period is mainly characterized by maturation of tissues and organs and rapid growth of body.

Growth in length is particularly striking during 3rd, 4th and 5th months.

Increase in weight is most striking during last 2 months (8th and 9th months) of gestation.

A few malformations also rise during fetal period mainly due to mechanical forces of intrauterine compression.

3rd month (9–12th weeks)

- Slow growth of head compared to rest body.
- Face is more human looking.
- Eyes come to lie ventrally and ears attain definitive position.

Limbs reach relative length due to development of primary centers of ossification around 12th week. External genitalia develops and sex of fetus can be determined in 3rd month (12 weeks).

4th and 5th months (16–20 weeks)

- Fetus is covered with fine hair known as lanugo. Hair visible in eyebrows and head.
- Fetus lengths rapidly.

Movements of fetus can be felt during 5th month (20 weeks) by mother → quickening.

6th month (24 weeks): Weight increases

Skin of fetus is reddish and wrinkled appearance because of lack of underlying connective tissue. Although several organs are able to function by 6th month; respiratory system and CNS have not differentiated sufficiently and coordination between the two systems not yet established. Fetus born during 6th month is difficult to survive.

7 to 8th month (28–32 weeks)

Skin covered with whitish fatty substance known as vernix caseosa composed of secretory products of sebaceous glands. Fetus obtains well rounded contours as a result of deposition of subcutaneous fat. Fetus born at 7th month (28 weeks) has 90% chance of surviving.

9th month (36–40 weeks)

Skull has largest circumference of all parts of body, an important fact → passage through birth canal. Sexual characteristics are more pronounced and testes in scrotum.

Date of birth is most accurately indicated as 266 days or 38 weeks after fertilization.

Obstetrician calculates date of birth as 280 days or 40 weeks from first day LNMP.

- Most of fetuses are born within 10–14 days of calculated delivered date.
- If they are born earlier → premature (32 weeks)
- If born later → postmature (42 weeks)
- Valuable tool for assisting the age determination is ultrasound.

Prenatal Screening Techniques for Prenatal Diagnosis

- Ultrasonography
- Amniocentesis
- Chorionic villus sampling.

Tests determine

1. Placental growth
2. Fetal growth
3. Congenital malformation
4. Chromosomal abnormalities.

Placenta: A Highly Vascular Organ

Human placenta is discoid, hemochorial and deciduate which connects the fetus with uterine wall of the mother. It is a fetomaternal organ that facilitates nutrition and gas exchange between maternal and fetal compartments.

Development of Human: Two Sources

1. *Fetal part:* Trophoblast and extraembryonic mesoderm → form chorionic frondosum.
2. *Maternal part* is uterine endometrium → decidua basalis.

Structure of placenta

At start of 4th month, placenta has two components:

1. Fetal part: Chorionic frondosum
2. Maternal part: Decidua basalis
   - On fetal side → placenta is bordered by chorionic plate
   - On the maternal side is decidua basalis (decidua plate).
   - Between chorionic plate and decidua plate are intervillous spaces filled with maternal blood lined by syncytium in which are floating villi.
   - Placental surface area is parallel to expanding uterus, throughout pregnancy.
   - Covers 15–30% of internal surface of uterus.
   - Full term placenta: Discoid, diameter 15–25 cm, 3 cm thick, weighs 500 to 600 gm

- At birth, torn from uterine wall, approximately 30 minutes after birth of the child and is expelled from the uterine cavity.

Two surfaces

1. Fetal surface covered by chorionic plate.
2. Maternal surface irregular with 15–30 cotyledons
   - Peripheral margin.

Placental barrier: It consists of tissues which intervene between blood in terminal villi and maternal blood in the intervillous space. Through this barrier exchange of gaseous and metabolites occur.

3rd month of pregnancy, placental barrier has 4 layers

1. Endothelium of fetal capillaries on the basement membrane.
2. Core of primary mesoderm.
3. Basement membrane of cytotrophoblast.
4. Syncytiotrophoblast

4th month onwards only 2 layers of placental membrane are seen

1. Endothelium of fetal capillaries.
2. Syncytiotrophoblast.
   Two layers form true placental barrier.

Functions of Placenta

1. Exchange of gases.
2. Exchange of nutrients and electrolytes.
3. Transmission of maternal antibodies.
4. Hormone production.
5. Placenta as an allograft with respect to mother.

TWINS AND FETAL MEMBRANES IN TWINS

Mother nurturing two conceptuses at the same time or single pregnancy is known as twinning.

Two types of twins

1. Monozygotic twins
2. Dizygotic twins

Arrangement of fetal membranes in twins varies considerably depending upon

1. Type of twins
2. Type of separation of monozygotic twins.

Dizygotic Twins or Fraternal Twins or Non-identical

1. Incidence of dizygotic increases with age of mother. Simultaneously shedding of two oocytes in single ovarian cycle either from one graafian follicle or two separate follicles and fertilization by two different spermatozoa at the same time. Two offspring born of the same pregnancy.
2. Twins derived from two zygotes.
3. Fraternal twins develop → in separate or partially fused chorionic and placenta and a separate amniotic sac.
4. Two zygotes have totally different genetic constitution, the twins have no resemblance.
5. They may or may not be of different sex.
6. Twins have no resemblance.
7. Both zygotes implant individually in the uterus and usually develop its own placenta, chorionic sac and amnion.
8. Sometimes two placentas are so close together, that they fuse.
9. Similarly, walls of chorionic sacs may also come close in apposition and fuse.
10. Separate amniotic sac.
11. Rarely each dizygotic twins possess red blood cells of two different types (erythrocyte mosaicism), indicating that fusion of two placentas was so intimate that RBCs have exchanged.

Monozygotic Twins or Identical Twins

Develop from single fertilization ovum. Incidence 3–4/1000 births. They result splitting of zygote at various stages of development. Earliest separation is to occur at 2 cells stage.

The fertilized egg gets divided into two embryos within 72 hours of conception, the two babies will develop in separate amniotic sacs.

1. Twins have strong resemblance, same sex, same blood group, fingerprints.
2. External appearance such as eye and hair color also resemble.

I. Separation at 2 cells stage

1. Separate zygote develop.
2. Both blastocysts implant separately and each embryo has its own placenta, chorionic sac and own amniotic cavity.

II. Splitting of zygote of inner cell mass (occurs at early blastocyst stage)

- Inner cell mass splits into two separate groups of cells within the same blastocyst cavity.
- Two embryos have common placenta and common chorionic cavity, but separate amniotic cavity.

III. In rare cases, separation occurs at still late at the bilaminar disc just before formation of primitive streak, i.e. splitting of inner cell mass at late stage

- Twins have single placenta, common chorion and amniotic sac.
- Though placenta is common, blood supply is usually well balanced.

Applied aspect

- Conjoined twins or siamese twins.
- Partial splitting of the primitive node and streak of the embryo. Classified according to nature and degree of union → thoracophagus, pygophagus or craniophagus.

- Occasionally monozygotic twins are connected by common skin bridge or common liver bridge.
  Many conjoined twins have survived.

Clinical Correlation

Twin pregnancy has high incidence of perinatal mortality and morbidity. 12% of twins are premature infants with low birth weight.

9

Development of CNS

BRAIN AND SPINAL CORD

Ectoderm germ cell layer gives rise to neural tube (CNS), i.e. brain and spinal cord by neurulation.

1. Neurulation includes the formation of:
   - Neural plate
   - Neural groove
   - Neural folds and fusion
   - Neural tube
   - Neural crest cells (give entire peripheral nervous system)
2. Starts during the late 3rd week (18th day)
3. Ends by the end of 4th week (28th day)
4. It is induced by the notochord.

Development of CNS appears at third week of IUL; as slipper shape plate of thickened ectoderm (neuroectoderm) neural plate or medullary plate, in mid-dorsal region of embryo in front of primitive node. With the formation of neuroectoderm, embryo is broader in cephalic than in caudal region. Under the inducing effect of the notochord (16th–22nd), the overlying neuroectoderm cells (neural tube epithelium) thickens to form the neural plate or medullary plate. Neural plate appears cranial to the primitive node and dorsal to notochord.

During somite period: 20–30th days or 3rd–4th week, lateral edges of neural plate become elevated to form neural folds and depression of mid-region forms neural groove. Tips of neural groove are lined by specialized cells. Neural crest cells, which are continuous with surface ectoderm. Neural folds approach each other in midline and fuse to neural tube. Fusion begins at cervical region or neck region (4th somite) and proceeds cranially and caudally except upper and lower ends. Once fusion is initiated the open ends of neural tube form neuropores. Cephalic or anterior neuropore and caudal or posterior neuropore communicate with amniotic cavity. neuropores provide nutrition to neural tube as blood vascular system is yet to develop. Closure of neuropores coincides with establishment of heart and blood vascular circulation which provides nutrition to developing neural tube.

Neurulation starts late 3rd week (18th day) and ends by the end of 4th week (28th day).

Neurulation is completed by 4th week. The cranial one-third of the neural tube represents the future brain and the caudal two-thirds represents the future spinal cord.

Broad end at cephalic region is characterized by dilations: Brain vesicles: Three types

1. Forebrain or prosencephalon
2. Midbrain or mesencephalon
3. Hindbrain or rhombencephalon.

Simultaneously cephalic end neural tube (brain)—two flexures develop

1. Cervical flexure → at junction of hindbrain and spinal cord.
2. Cephalic flexure → in midbrain region.

5th week prosencephalon consists of two parts

a. Telencephalon has two lateral outpocking → right and left cerebral hemispheres.
b. Diencephalon with outgrowth optic vesicles.

Rhombencephalon also consists of two parts

A. Metencephalon → forms pons and cerebellum.

B. Myelencephalon → medulla oblongata

- Boundary between these two portions is marked by pontine flexure.
- Cavity of spinal cord is central canal continuous with that of brain vesicles (CSF)
- Cavity of rhombencephalon → IV ventricle
- Cavity of diencephalon → III ventricle
- Cerebral hemispheres → lateral ventricle
- Lumen of mesencephalon is narrow aqueduct of Sylvius connects III and IV ventricles.
- Position of spinal cord

3rd month (IUL) spinal cord occupies entire length of vertebral canal.

At birth, spinal cord is at the level of 3rd lumbar vertebra.

At puberty reaches final position, opposite intervertebral disc between 1st and 2nd lumbar vertebrae.

Cervical and lumbar enlargements of spinal cord appear 5th or 6th week of IUL with development of upper and lower buds.

Cranial Nerves and Their Functional Components

Cranial Nerves—12 Pairs

    I. Olfactory nerve—sensory.

    II. Optic nerve—sensory.

    III. Oculomotor nerve—motor.

    IV. Trochlear nerve—motor

    V. Trigeminal nerve—mixed.

    VI. Abducent nerve—motor.

    VII. Facial nerve—mixed.

VIII. Vestibulocochlear nerve—sensory.

    IX. Glossopharyngeal nerve—mixed.

    X. Vagus nerve—mixed.

XI. Accessory nerve—motor

XII. Hypoglossal nerve—motor

Basal plate → contains motor nuclei and divided into 3 groups, is ventromedial.

Alar plate → contains 4 groups of sensory nuclei, is dorso-lateral.

Basal and alar plates are separated by sulcus limitans.

Arrangement of neurons in brainstem (medulla, pons and midbrain)

Alar lamina gives rise to sensory neurons and basal lamina gives rise to motor neurons which form the nuclei of cranial nerves.

In brainstem the motor and sensory neurons are basically organized in longitudinal columns.

Cranial nerve nuclei in the brainstem are arranged in 7 longitudinal columns. Functional components of CN nuclei.

Efferent neurons (derived from basal lamina) are arranged medial to lateral (3 longitudinal columns)

1. Somatic efferent (SE) column—III, IV, VI and XII (striated muscles)
2. Special visceral efferent (SpVE) column—V, VII, IX, X and XI.
3. General visceral efferent (GVE) column—III, VII, IX and X. Cranial part of preganglionic parasympathetic outflow.

Afferent neurons (derived from alar lamina) are arranged medial to lateral side in 4 longitudinal columns

4. General visceral afferent: X (viscera)
5. Special visceral afferent: VII, IX and X (gustatory)
6. General somatic afferent (GSA): V (exteroceptive, proprioceptive)
7. Special somatic afferent (SpSA): VIII (hearing and balancing)

Functional Components of CN Nuclei

1. Oculomotor nuclei: SE and GVE
2. Trochlear nuclei: SE
3. Trigeminal nuclei: GSA and SpVE
4. Abducent nuclei: SE
5. Facial nerve nuclei: SpVE, GVE, SpVA and GSA
6. Vestibular and cochlear nuclei: SpSA (I and II CN→ SpSA)
7. Glossopharyngeal nuclei: SpVE, GVE, GVA and SpVA
8. Vagus nerve nuclei: SpVE, GVE, GVA, SpVA and GSA
9. Accessory nerve nuclei: SpVE
10. Hypoglossal nerve nuclei: SE.

10

Embryology of the Eyeball

Eye develops from 3 sources

- Neuroectoderm of forebrain.
- Surface ectoderm of head region.
- Mesoderm (mesenchyme) between neuroectoderm of forebrain and surface ectoderm of head region, i.e. neural crest cells.

Rudiments of eye appear 4th week before the closure of anterior neuropore (25th day). In form of 2 lateral diverticulae from lateral wall of diencephalon.

Appear as a pair of shallow grooves to optic grooves (sulci) on side of forebrain.

22nd day of conception optic grooves form optic peduncles. These peduncles are bilateral evagination of neuroectoderm of the forebrain. With closure of neural tube these grooves form outpockings of the forebrain. Optic peduncles distally form optic vesicles. Optic vesicles connected to forebrain by hollow stalk, optic stalk with forebrain.

Optic vesicles come in contact with surface ectoderm and induce changes in the surface ectoderm to thicken to formation of lens placodes.

Optic vesicle dilates and invaginates and sinks below surface ectoderm, and forms double walled optic cup.

Optic cup has inner and outer layers initially separated by a lumen, the intraretinal space.

Invagination of optic vesicle is not restricted to central portion of the cup but also involves part of the inferior surface that forms choroid fissure, through hyaloid artery and vein reaches the inner chamber of eye.

During the 7th week (50th day) of IUL, lips of choroid fissure fuse and mouth of optic cup becomes round opening future pupil. Rim of optic cup becomes iris.

Optic cup: Inner layer forms neuroepithelium→"neural retina".

Outer layer forms retinal pigment epithelium. Cavity of optic stalk → axons of ganglion cells → optic nerve.

Eye Development

1. Retina → optic vesicle—optic cup from forebrain (neural tube), i.e. neuroectoderm outer layer forms pigment layer and inner layer forms multilaminar neural layer of retina.
2. Sclera and choroid → loose mesenchyme (neural crest cells) surround optic cup.
3. Sphincter and dilator pupillae and ciliary muscle → neuroectoderm and NCC (iris and ciliary body).
4. Lens → lens vesicle → surface ectoderm
5. Cornea → surface ectoderm (outer epithelium), stroma and inner epithelium → mesenchyme (NCC).
6. Conjunctiva → surface ectoderm.

Development of Ear

Ear has 3 parts: External ear, middle ear and internal ear.

External ear develops from first pharyngeal cleft (ectoderm). External ear has 3 parts: Auricle, external acoustic (auditory) meatus) and eardrum.

Middle ear develops from first pharyngeal pouch (endoderm). 3 ossicles, 2 muscles, nerves and blood vessels lie in petrous bone.

Internal ear develops from otic placode (surface ectoderm) and neural crest cells. 3 semicircular canals (3 semicircular duct) and vestibule (macula and saccule) and cochlea (cochlear duct).

Function: External ear sound collecting organ. Middle ear sound conductor from external ear to internal ear.

Internal ear converts sound waves into nerve impulses and registers changes in equilibrium,which conveyed to brain by VIII cranial nerve.

Internal Ear Development

First indication of developing ear in embryo is at about 22nd day (3rd week). Thickening of surface ectoderm on each side of rhombencephalon, the otic placodes.

Otic placodes invaginate rapidly and form otic or auditory pits get separated from surface ectoderm form otic or auditory vesicle (otocysts).

Otic vesicle forms membranous labyrinth: It forms the neuroepithelium of cochlear duct (hearing) and 3 semicircular ducts, utricle and saccule and ganglions (spiral and vestibular).

Mesenchyme derived from neural crest cells surrounding cochlear duct differentiates into cartilage. Otic capsule that forms bony cochlea.

Middle Ear Development

From the 1st pharyngeal pouch (IPP) and dorsal part of 2nd pharyngeal pouch (endoderm) that form the tubotympanic recess. Distal part of tubotympanic recess widen to form primitive tympanic cavity (middle ear) and proximal part narrow to form auditory tube which communicates with nasopharynx. It also forms inner mucous lining of tympanic membrane.

Ossicles: Malleus and incus are derived from 1st pharyngeal arch (PA) and stapes is derived from 2nd pharyngeal arch. Supporting ligaments of ossicles develop later.

Muscles: Tensor tympani derived from 1st PA supplied by mandibular nerve and stapedius from 2nd PA supplied by facial nerve.

Middle ear attains adult size at birth.

External Ear Development

External acoustic meatus develops from 1st pharyngeal cleft (PC).

Eardrum or tympanic membrane: 3 germ layers

1. Ectoderm epithelial lining (outside) → cuticle layer of 1st PC.
2. Endodermal epithelial lining of the tympanic cavity, inner → mucous layer of IPP.
3. Intermediate layer of connective tissue (mesoderm) forms the fibrous layer.

Auricle: Develops from 6 mesenchymal portions at dorsal ends of 1st and 2nd PAs surrounding the 1st PC.

Clinical Correlates: Deafness and External Ear Abnormalities

Congenital deafness, usually associated mutism:

1. Abnormal development of the membranous and bony labyrinths.
2. Malformations of the auditory ossicles and eardrum.
3. Extreme cases, the tympanic cavity and external acoustic meatus are absent.
    - Most forms of congenital deafness are caused genetic factors.
    - Environmental factors may also interfere with normal development of the internal and middle ears.
    - Rubella virus, affecting the embryo in the 7 or 8 weeks, may cause severe damage to the organ of Corti.

Erythroblastosis fetalis, diabetes, hypothyroidism and toxoplasmosis can cause congenital deafness.

12

Branchial Apparatus

BRANCHIAL ARCHES

Branchial apparatus consists of branchial (pharyngeal) arches which are mesodermal, branchial (pharyngeal) pouches which are endodermal and branchial (pharyngeal) clefts which are ectodermal closely related to primitive pharynx.

Pharyngeal or Branchial Arches 6—Pairs Appear around 4th and 5th Weeks of IU

Most typical feature of head and neck is formed by branchial arches which contribute for external appearance of embryo. Branchial arches—6 pairs of cylindrical mesodermal bars extend from hindbrain region. 5th pair is rudimentary. They contribute to formation of neck and face, definitive mouth, pharynx and larynx.

Pharyngeal or branchial arches are separated by deep ectodermal clefts, i.e. pharyngeal clefts (4 pairs), external and internal arches are separated by pharyngeal pouches (4 pairs).

Each pharyngeal arch covered outside by surface ectoderm and inside lined by endodermal epithelium of pharyngeal gut and consists mesodermal core.

Each pharyngeal arch is characterized by

1. Own muscle component.
2. Own cranial nerve.
3. Skeletal component.
4. An arterial component.

I. Pharyngeal Arch: Skeletal Component

1. Dorsal portion is maxillary process which extends beneath eye and forms premaxilla, maxilla, zygomatic and part of temporal bone via membranous ossification.
   Maxillary process forms the upper lip, upper jaw, palate.
2. Ventral portion → mandibular process contains Meckel's cartilage.
   a. Meckel's cartilage disappears except at the dorsal end persists to form malleus and incus (middle ear ossicles).
   b. Anterior ligament of malleus and sphenomandibular ligament.
   c. Mandible is formed by membranous ossification from mesenchyme surrounding Meckel's cartilage.

Muscle component of 1st arch (8 muscles)

1. Muscles of mastication → temporalis, lateral and medial pterygoid and masseter.
2. Anterior belly of digastric and mylohyoid (suprahyoid muscles)
3. Tensor tympani and tensor veli palatini.
   Nerve supply is mandibular nerve, branch of trigeminal nerve (5th cranial nerve).
   All muscles migrate from the skeletal element except tensor tympani attached to malleus.

II. Pharyngeal Arch or Hyoid Arch: Reichert Cartilage

Skeletal component is known as Reichert cartilage. It extends dorsally up to ear capsule.

1. Dorsal part → stapes of middle ear, succeeding part forms styloid process of temporal bone and stylohyoid ligament.
2. Ventral part → lesser cornu and upper part of hyoid bone.

Muscles of 2nd Arch: Innervations by Facial Nerve

1. Muscles of facial expression include epicranius and platysma.

2. Auricular muscles.
3. Posterior belly of digastric and stylohyoid.
4. Stapedius → which is attached to skeletal component.

III. Pharyngeal Arch

Skeletal component:

1. Ventral part forms greater cornu and lower part of body of hyoid bone.
2. Dorsal part → disappears.

Muscle component of 3rd arch: Nerve supply is glossopharyngeal nerve (9th cranial nerve). 3rd PA has only one muscle, the stylopharyngeus.

5th pharyngeal arch is transitory.

4th and 6th Pharyngeal Arches

Skeletal component

4th pharyngeal arch ventral part is thyroid cartilage.

6th pharyngeal arch ventral part is cricoid, arytenoids, corniculate and cuneiform cartilages.

Dorsal parts of 4th and 6th arches disappear.

Muscle component of 4th and 6th arches

1. 4th pharyngeal arch is cricothyroid muscle supplied by external laryngeal nerve, branch of superior laryngeal nerve (vagus X cranial nerve).
2. 6th pharyngeal arch→ all intrinsic muscles of larynx supplied by recurrent laryngeal nerve (cranial accessory nerve via vagus).

Pharyngeal Pouches (Endodermal)

Primordial pharynx derived from the foregut. It widens cranially where it joins the stomadeum and narrows caudally where it joins esophagus. Its lateral wall presents evaginations which are pharyngeal pouches.

Endodermal derivatives of pharyngeal gut grouped in 2 broad divisions

1. Ventral derivatives developing from the floor of primitive pharynx (tongue).
2. Lateral derivatives are evaginations, the pharyngeal pouches.

PP is numbered craniocaudal direction. In human embryo has 4 pairs and 5th rudimentary pharyngeal pouch.

Ventral derivatives from floor of primitive pharynx that is the cranial part of foregut (dorsal) form

1. Tongue rudiment.
2. Thyroid diverticulum
3. Laryngotracheal groove that gives lower respiratory system.

Lateral derivatives: Pharyngeal pouches have 4 pairs. Each pharyngeal pouch has two parts—the ventral part and the dorsal part. Ventral part of each pouch is obliterated by the developing tongue rudiment. Dorsal part of each pouch except for first is divided into ventral and dorsal wings.

Dorsal part of the 1st pharyngeal pouch (no ventral or dorsal wings)

Dorsal part of 1st pouch forms a stalk → diverticulum, tubotympanic recess and comes in contact with 1st pharyngeal cleft (ectodermal) and forms external acoustic meatus.

Medial is the proximal part remains tubular or narrow forms eustachian or auditory tube which communicates with nasopharynx.

Lateral (distal part) widens into a sac like forms primitive tympanic cavity (middle ear) and mastoid antrum.

1. Mucous lining of middle ear, mastoid antrum and mastoid air cells
2. Inner lining of tympanic membrane.
3. Auditory tube.

Dorsal part of the 2nd pharyngeal pouch

It has two parts:

1. Dorsal wing of 2nd pharyngeal pouch joins 1st pharyngeal pouch and contributes for tubotympanic recess.
2. Ventral wing: Palatine tonsil that communicates with oropharynx.

2nd pharyngeal pouch (ventral wing)

1. Endoderm of 2nd PP forms stratified squamous non-keratinized epithelium lining of tonsillar crypts on pharyngeal or medial surface of tonsil.
2. Mesoderm forms lymphatic tissue, fibrous capsule and connective tissue of tonsil.
3. Remnants of pouch: Intratonsillar cleft.

Dorsal part of the 3rd pharyngeal pouch

It has two parts:

1. Dorsal wing forms epithelium of inferior parathyroid gland (parathyroid III)
2. Ventral wing forms thymus gland.

Dorsal part of 4th pharyngeal pouch

1. Dorsal wing forms superior parathyroid gland (parathyroid IV)
2. Ventral wing joins 5th rudimentary pharyngeal pouch and forms caudal pharyngeal complex gives rise to 3 structures.

Dorsal part of 5th pharyngeal pouch

It is last to develop and joins the ventral wing of 4th pharyngeal pouch and it forms caudal pharyngeal complex.

Caudal pharyngeal complex: It has 3 structures:

1. *Thymic part* incorporated into developing thymus.
2. *Lateral thyroid rudiment* fuses with median thyroid rudiment (derived from thyroglossal duct) induces the differentiation of thyroid gland.
3. Ultimobrachial body → C cells of thyroid gland (parafollicular cells → calcitonin)

Pharyngeal Clefts or Grooves Develop around 5th Week

Embryo is characterized by presence of 4 pharyngeal clefts of which only the first contributes for definitive structure of embryo. There are invaginations of surface ectoderm between pharyngeal arches.

1st pharyngeal cleft forms

1. External acoustic meatus
2. Cuticle layer of tympanic membrane.

Active proliferation of mesenchymal tissue in 2nd arch overlaps the 3rd and 4th arches and obliterates clefts 2, 3 and 4 and loose contact with outside. With further development smooth concavity of side of definitive neck is restored.

13

Development of Endocrines

DEVELOPMENT OF SUPRARENAL GLANDS

Each gland consists of two components: External cortex and internal medulla, which have different embryonic origins.

Cortex is derived from the mesothelium (coelomic epithelium: Mesoderm) lining the posterior abdominal wall. The cortex is formed of two parts:

1. Thick fetal cortex
2. Thin layer of cells that will later form the adult cortex.

Differentiation of suprarenal cortical zones begins during the late fetal period.

Zona glomerulosa and zona fasciculata are present at birth. Zona reticularis, is not recognizable until the end of third year. After birth, fetal cortex starts rapid degeneration and vanishes totally during the first year of life. Adult cortex starts to proliferate becomes fully differentiated by the 12th year.

Adrenal cortex poorly developed in anencephalic fetuses

Medulla: It forms a mass medial to the fetal cortex and derived from neural crest cells (ectoderm) and from adjacent sympathetic ganglion. While the fetal cortex is being formed, cells originating in the sympathetic system of the neural crest cells invade its medial aspect, where they are arranged in cords and clusters. Cells that give rise to medulla and stain yellowish brown with chrome salts and hence called chromaffin cells. During embryonic life chromaffin cells are scattered widely throughout the embryo. But in adult chromaffin cells are seen only in medulla of adrenal gland.

Applied: Suprarenal glands rapidly become smaller during the first 2–3 weeks after birth, due to the rapid regression of the fetal cortex.

Its involution completed in the first year of life.

During the process of involution, the cortex is friable and susceptible to trauma leading to severe hemorrhage.

Development of Thyroid Gland—4th Week

Thyroid gland appears as endodermal epithelial proliferation from the floor of pharynx between tuberculum impar and copula of His which is indicated as foramen caecum. It forms median thyroid rudiment, the thyroglossal duct (endodermal).

Thyroglossal duct descends in front of pharyngeal gut ventral to hyoid bone and laryngeal cartilages. It reaches final position in front of trachea by 7th week. Tip of it forms bilobed mass the two lateral lobes with small median isthmus.

Caudal pharyngeal complex

1. Lateral thyroid rudiment joins median thyroid rudiment and induces the differentiation of development of gland.
2. Parafollicular cells derived from ultimobranchial body (5th pharyngeal pouch) are incorporated into gland a source for calcitonin.

Thyroid begins to function, 3rd month of IUL → thyroxin

Neural crest cells invade and form connective tissue and capsule.

Subsequently thyroglossal duct disappears. Cephalic end is foramen caecum of tongue. Caudal end of duct is pyramidal lobe attached to isthmus.

Development of Pituitary Gland or Hypophysis Cerebri

It has two complete parts

A. *Anterior pituitary (adenohypophysis):* Ectodermal outpocking (upward) of stomadeum (primitive oral cavity) immediately in front of oropharyngeal membrane known as Rathke's pouch.

B. *Posterior pituitary (neurohypophysis)* Neuroectoderm, a downward extension of diencephalon, the infundibulum.

Anterior pituitary—3 weeks: Rathke's pouch appears as evagination of oral cavity from roof of stomadeum in front of oropharyngeal membrane and cranial end of notochord. Rathke's pouch subsequently grows dorsally towards the floor of forebrain vesicle and in contact with infundibulum. By end of 2nd month it loses its connection with oral cavity and comes close contact with infundibulum.

Cephalic part of Rathke's pouch forms anterior pituitary or adenohypophysis

1. Anterior wall of Rathke's pouch increases rapidly and forms pars distalis or pars anterior.
2. Small extension of this lobe grows along the stalk of infundibulum and eventually surrounds it and forms pars tuberculum.
3. Posterior wall of Rathke's pouch develops into pars intermedia. In human it has a little significance. It embraces the posterior lobe.
4. Cavity of pouch persists as after birth as intraglandular cleft.

Posterior pituitary or neurohypophysis

Funnel-shaped diverticulum grows caudally from the floor of diencephalon (neuroectoderm).

It lies close to dorsal surface of cephalic part of Rathke's pouch → infundibulum.

Infundibulum (Neuroectoderm)

1. Lower end of infundibulum forms pars nervosa (posterior lobe) of hypophysis cerebri.
2. Stem forms infundibulum stalk.
3. Upper end forms median eminence.
4. Cavity persists as infundibulum recess of 3rd ventricle.

Clinical Correlation

Position of commencement of Rathke's pouch corresponds where nasal septum meets the palate. Bony craniopharyngeal canal is occasionally present in the floor of hypophyseal fossa of sphenoid bone which indicates remnant of Rathke's pouch.

14

Development of Tongue: Floor of Primitive Pharynx

Tongue appears 4th week and derived from 3 parts

1. Mucous membrane → endoderm of the primitive pharynx.
2. Fibroareolar tissue → mesoderm of pharyngeal arches.
3. Muscles → occipital myotomes.

Development of tongue

I. Small median swelling → tuberculum impar
   Two oval lateral swellings → lingual swellings
II. Caudal to tuberculum impar, another median endodermal elevation is the hypobranchial eminence or copula of His.

Three endodermal elevations are formed due to proliferation of underlying mesenchyme

1. Small median swelling → tuberculum impar. Unpaired between 1st and 2nd pharyngeal arches.
2. Two oval lateral swellings → lingual swellings (a pair at ventral end of 1st pharyngeal arch).

   These swellings appear before the ventral ends of 1st and 2nd pharyngeal arches meet their opposite side.

   Two lingual swellings grow and increase in size, later over grow into tuberculum impar and emerge with one another and form a combine mass and form → a two-thirds of tongue or oral part. It forms body of tongue which bilateral in origin.

   Caudal to median tongue bud (tuberculum impar), another median endodermal elevation is the hypobranchial eminence or copula of His. It is contributed by ventral ends of 2nd, 3rd and 4th arches which converge.

A transverse groove separates

- Caudal part → forms epiglottis
- Cranial part → forms posterior one-third of tongue (pharyngeal part). It mainly contributed by 3rd arch.
- Line of fusion between anterior two-thirds and posterior one-third is V-shaped sulcus terminalis, apex is foramen caecum.

MUCOUS MEMBRANE: ENDODERM OF PHARYNX

1. Muscles of tongue from occipital myotomes, which migrate and invade tongue rudiment in floor of mouth. Migration of occipital myotomes drags the 12th cranial nerve or hypoglossal nerve.
2. Fibroareolar part is mesoderm of 1st, 2nd and 3rd pharyngeal arches which bind the tongue muscles.

Composite development of tongue explains its sensory nerve (4) supply

1. Mucous membrane of anterior two-thirds from interphalangeal arch.
   i. General sensation is lingual nerve → branch of mandibular nerve (post-trematic nerve)
   ii. Special sensation is chorda tympani nerve → branch of facial nerve (pre-trematic nerve)
2. Mucous membrane of posterior one-third of tongue originates 3rd pharyngeal arch. General and special sensation nerve is glossopharyngeal nerve.
3. Most posterior part of tongue (root) and epiglottis derived from 4th pharyngeal arch. General and special sensation is superior laryngeal nerve (vagus).
4. Muscles of tongue → hypoglossal nerve (12th cranial nerve) except palatoglossus (cranial nerve XI).

Anomalies of Tongue

Aglossia completes absence of tongue rudiment.
Hemiglossia—suppression of one of lingual swelling.

15

Development of Face:
4–12th Weeks

Development of face is around stomadeum. It is contributed by 5 facial prominences consisting of neural crest derived mesenchyme. Mainly contributed by first pair of pharyngeal arches.

1. Maxillary processes → lateral to stomadeum
2. Mandibular processes → caudal to stomadeum
   These are 1st pharyngeal arches.
3. Frontonasal process → formed by proliferation of mesenchyme ventral to forebrain vesicle constitutes the upper border of stomadeum.

Face of embryo is recognized by 5 mesenchymal prominences

A. Unpaired frontonasal prominences: Rounded elevation, cranial to stomadeum.
B. Pair of maxillary prominences: It is dorsal part of 1st pharyngeal arch, lateral to stomadeum.
C. Pair of mandibular prominences: It is ventral part of 1st pharyngeal arch, caudal to stomadeum.

5th week: On both sides of frontonasal prominences, local thickenings on surface ectoderm are nasal placodes (olfactory).

Nasal placodes invaginate deep into underlying mesenchyme to form nasal pits. Each pit is surrounded by two nasal prominences.

Along the outer edge is lateral nasal prominence and along medial edge is medial nasal prominence.

Mandibular prominences are first to fuse along the lower border of stomadeum and form the lower jaw and lower lip.

Two maxillary processes compressing medial nasal prominences. Subsequently cleft between medial nasal prominences and maxillary processes is lost and both fuse to form upper lip.

Lateral nasal prominences do not participate in formation of upper lip.

Development of Nose is Formed 5 Prominences

Frontal nasal prominences form bridge of nose.

Merged medial nasal prominences (globular process forms crest and tip of nose).

Lateral nasal prominences form the side of nose (ala).

Fusion of maxillary prominence and mandibular prominence forms the oral fissure (opening of mouth). Excessive fusion causes microstomia, less or non-fusion causes macrostomia.

The mesenchyme from the 1st and 2nd pairs of pharyngeal arches invade the facial prominences

1. Muscles of mastication
2. Muscles of facial expression.

Embryological basis of sensory innervations of the face

1. Area derived from the frontonasal process is supplied by ophthalmic nerve (V1).
2. Area derived from the maxillary process is supplied by maxillary nerve (V2).
3. Area derived from the mandibular process is supplied by mandibular nerve (V2).

DEVELOPMENT OF PALATE: 5–10 WEEKS

Begins at the 5th week completed by 12th week.

The most critical period for the development of palate is from 6 to 9th weeks.

Palate develops from 2 primordia.

Primary Palate and Secondary Palate

Primary Palate

1. Formation of medial nasal prominences → derived frontonasal prominence.
2. Fusion of medial nasal prominences (MNPs) → globular process.
3. Formation of intermaxillary segment.

Palatal component forms the primary palate, which becomes future premaxilla bearing 4 incisor teeth.

Secondary Palate

Secondary palate is formed by 2 shelf-like outgrowth from inner part of maxillary prominences palatine shelves or plates (6th week). Secondary palate—fuse each other, posterior part of the primary palate and above with nasal septum.

Fusion with the nasal septum begins anteriorly at 9th week, extends posteriorly and is completed by 12th week.

Fusion of secondary palate (palatine shelves) with primary palate→ definitive palate.

Bone develops: Anterior part to form the hard palate.

Posterior part develops as muscular soft palate.

The primary palate represents only a small part lying anterior to the incisive fossa, of the adult hard palate.

Applied: Cleft lip coupled with clefts of the anterior palate or entire palate.

16

Introduction to Embryology of Cardiovascular System

Vascular system in human embryo appears in the 3rd week of IUL, when embryo is no longer able to satisfy its nutritional requirements by diffusion alone.

Three Stages

1. Nutrition of embryo in early stage of development.
2. Development of extraembryonic blood vascular system.
3. Development of intraembryonic blood vascular system and heart.

Blood vascular system is formed by 3rd week of IUL in 2 stages.

Development of extraembryonic blood vascular system: Early part of 3rd week of development: Blood vessels develop from angioblasts which differentiate from mesenchyme of 3 regions: (1) Wall of yolk sac; (2) connecting stalk; (3) chorion.

Capillary plexuses of the yolk sac form vitelline vessels. Capillary plexuses of chorion and umbilical stalk form umbilical vessels. Extraembryonic vessels gradually penetrate the embryo proper and become continuous with intraembryonic blood vascular system.

Development of intraembryonic vessels and heart occurs in mesoderm-II germ layer in the later part of 3rd week development.

Intraembryonic blood vessels develop as cell clusters at first, on the lateral sides of the embryo, soon spread rapidly in a cephalic direction they acquire a lumen, unite and form a plexus of small blood vessels becomes horseshoe-shaped → primitive heart tube.

In addition, clusters of angiogenetic cells appear bilaterally and parallel and close to the midline of the embryonic area. Acquire a lumen and form a pair of longitudinal vessels, the *dorsal aortae*. At a later date, connect up with the horseshoe-shaped plexus (the heart tube). Caudally end embryonic area the two dorsal aortas extend into connecting stalk as umbilical arteries, which break up into capillaries of chorionic villi.

Returning venules from the chorion join to form umbilical veins (oxygenated blood) in the connecting stalk. Each umbilical veins run cranially in the embryo towards primitive tube.

Capillary plexuses within the yolk sac form vitelline vessels. Capillary plexuses of chorion and umbilical stalk form umbilical vessels. Cardinal veins which drain embryo's body wall also negotiate and join the primitive heart tube.

Primitive cardiovascular system: Primitive heart tube: Paired by the 4th week, fuses craniocaudal.

Arteries

1. Dorsal aortae
2. Vitelline arteries
3. Umbilical arteries
4. Aortic arch: 6 pairs

Veins

1. Common cardinal vein (anterior cardinal vein and posterior cardinal vein)
2. Vitelline veins
3. Umbilical veins

17

Development of Heart Tube

Vascular system appears in middle of 3rd week and completed by end of 8th week of gestation. Cardiac progenitor cells lie in epiblast immediate lateral to primitive streak. They migrate through primitive streak to proceed cranially. With time form horseshoe-shaped endothelial lined tube known as cardiogenic area. Cardiogenic plate intervenes between dorsal wall of yolk sac and floor of splanchnic pleuric mesoderm of pericardial cavity.

Cells migrate between ectoderm and endoderm and arrange longitudinal cellular strands → cardiogenic cords. Cords become canalized to form two thin walled → 2 endocardial heart tubes. Horseshoe-shaped endothelial tube surrounded myoblasts → also derived from splanchnopleuric mesoderm. Longitudinal bilateral parallel blood islands form dorsal aortae join cardiac area. As a result cephalocaudal and lateral folds (due to rapid growth of neural tube and somites) of paired cardiac primordia merge except in caudal part.

Formation of single heart tube—22nd–24th days (4th week)

As lateral folds occur endocardial heart tubes gradually approach each other and fuse from cephalocaudal direction to form single unpaired heart tube. Initially heart tube lies ventral to pericardial cavity with cranial folds and lateral folds heart tube comes dorsal to pericardial cavity. The fused heart now enters through dorsal wall pericardial cavity.

Fusion of heart tubes is followed by fusion of pericardial cavity.

Fusion of the heart tube is completed by 22nd–24th days, followed by ventral migration of heart. Heart tube enters the pericardial cavity and attached dorsally by dorsal mesocardium.

But heart tube firmly fixed at 2 sites, an arterial end (cranial) and venous end (caudal). No ventral mesocardium. Heart starts to beat on the 22nd day.

Paired endothelial heart tube initially in cervical region then descends to the thorax with the development of neck. With the head fold the pericardial cavity and heart undergoes 180 degrees rotation.

Two tubes separated by pericardial cavity by thick mesodermal tissue → myoepicardial mantle (that forms myocardium and epicardium).

It receives venous blood at caudal pole, and begins the pump blood out first aortic arch into dorsal aorta at its cranial pole.

Intraembryonic mesoderm cranial to the cardiogenic area forms the septum transversum.

Cephalocaudal fold, it comes to lie first ventral to pericardial cavity → finally caudal to heart tube. Septum transversum forms diaphragm separates thoracic cavity from abdominal cavity.

Cardiogenic area (primitive heart tube) is bounded

- Ventrally → pericardial sac
- Dorsally → foregut.
- Cephalically→ stomadeum and buccopharyngeal membrane.
- Caudally → septum transversum

Wall of heart tube

Myoepicardial mantle differentiates:
1. Outer epicardium (visceral pericardium)
2. Inner cells differentiate into myoblasts which form myocardium of heart.
3. Innermost endothelial tube forms endocardium of heart.

Paired Cardiac Primordia Form the Heart Tube

1. Consisting of inner endocardium (endothelial layer)
2. Myoepicardial mantle forms myocardium and epicardium (visceral layer of serous pericardium), which also forms coronary arteries.
3. Parietal layer of serous pericardium→ somatopleuric layer of pericardial cavity.

Mesothelial cells from septum transversum migrate over epicardium and form fibrous pericardium.

Longitudinal heart tube exhibits externally four circular constrictions which divide the tube into 5 saccular intercommunicating dilations.

These sacculations caudocranially are

1. Sinus venous
2. Primitive atrium
3. Primitive ventricle
4. Bulbus cordis
5. Truncus arteriosus.

Sinus venosus presents right and left horns and plunges into septum transversum.

Truncus arteriosus is ventral aorta connected to dorsal aorta by 5 pairs of aortic arches.

Each horn of sinus venosus receives 3 pairs of veins

A. Vitelline veins from yolk sac
B. Umbilical veins from placenta
C. Common cardinal veins (duct of Cuvier) from body wall.

Vitelline veins and umbilical veins traverse through septum transversum.

18

Formation of Cardiac Loop: 24 to 28th Days (4th Week)

Cardiac primordia develops 3rd week (16–18th days). Migration or fusion of two endothelial heart tubes is completed by 22–24th days. Heart starts beating as early as 24th day. Blood enters via the caudal part of heart tube and leaves through cranial end. Heart is suspended in the pericardial cavity by blood vessels at cranial and caudal poles. Endothelial heart tube connected dorsal by dorsal mesocardium.

1. Cranial end of single tube is arterial end of heart and it bifurcates into 2 branches known as aortic sac or ventral aorta with right and left horns.

2. Horns of ventral aorta are now connected to bilateral dorsal aorta with 6 pairs of aortic arch arteries.

3. Ventral aorta is now connected to dorsal aorta with aortic arch arteries which pass by side of foregut (pharynx) and become continuous with dorsal aorta.

4. Caudal end of single heart tube is venous end of heart is embedded in septum transversum and presents right and left horns. Each horn of sinus venosus receives 3 pairs of veins:

   A. Vitelline veins from yolk sac.

   B. Umbilical veins from placenta.

   C. Common cardinal veins (duct of Cuvier) from body wall.

Formation of cardiac loop between 23rd and 28th days

Heart tube continuous to elongate as cells are added from SHF to its cranial end.

The lengthening process is essential for the formation of out flow tracts → conus cordis and truncus arteriosus → ascending aorta and pulmonary trunk and it results in looping.

The primitive tube elongates within the pericardial cavity. Bulbus cordis and ventricle grow more rapidly than atrium and sinsus venosus (SV). With the result heart tube bends ventrally into pericardial cavity → 24th day (U and then S), the cardiac loop. This bend is cardiac loop which is completed by 28th day. Bulbus cordis and ventricle are in pericardial cavity. Later the atrium and the SV which outside also enter the pericardial cavity. The heart tube elongates towards the right side. Looping becomes the first visual sign of left–right asymmetry of the body.

Cephalic limb of loop → occupied by bulbus cordis and truncus arteriosus (outflow tract of ventricle, i.e. aorta and pulmonary trunk).

Primitive ventricle lies at summit or apex of loop.

Caudal limb of loop is primitive atrium and sinus venosus.

Cephalic portion of the tube bends in ventral, caudal and to the right. Caudal portion (atrial) shifts in dorsocranial and to the left. While cardiac looping is forming, local expansions become visible throughout the length of the heart tube. Atrium lies dorsal and slightly to left of common bulboventricular cavity and it is free from septum transversum. The atrial chamber and sinus venosus also get incorporated in pericardial cavity freed from septum transversum.

Atrial chamber grows transversely lies behind truncus arteriosus and expands. It projects forwards on either side of TA → auricles. Primitive atrium initially two, fuses as it and become single primitive atrial chamber as it enters pericardial cavity and dorsal to truncus arteriosus.

The sinus venosus is dorsal to primitive atrium and also shifted from septum transversum and remain double structure with 2 horns.

Each horn receives 3 important veins

1. Vitelline or omphalomesenteric veins from yolk sac.
2. Umbilical veins carry oxygenated blood from placenta (lateral to vitelline veins).
3. Common cardinal veins (duct of Cuvier) from the cephalic (ACV) and caudal (PCV) parts of body wall.

Sinus venosus ventrally communicates with primitive atrium chamber. At first communication between sinus venosus and atrium is wide. Soon entrance shifted to the right of primitive atrium → sinuatrial orifice. Bulbo-ventricular loop is initially suspended from dorsal wall of pericardial cavity by dorsal mesocardium.

With continuous growth of cardiac loop, dorsal mesocardium ruptures forming transverse sinus which is between arterial (BC and V) and venous ends (atrium) of U tube.

External atrioventricular junction is wide, but internal AV junction remains narrow as atrioventricular canal.

The junction between primitive ventricle and bulbus cordis, externally as bulboventricular sulcus, it is primary IVF. Subsequent changes in the development lead to formation of septation of various chambers of heart and which takes place simultaneously in next 4 weeks (5–8 weeks of IUL). At the end of cardiac looping → 24–28th days.

Definitive heart, the wall formed 24–28th days

1. Endocardium → endothelial heart tube.
2. Myocardium → myoepicardial mantle.
3. Epicardium → visceral layer of serous pericardium

4. Parietal layer of serous pericardium → somatopleuric layer of pericardial sac.
5. Fibrous pericardium → septum transversum.

Definitive Heart Tube

1. Primordium of cardiac plate → 16th day
2. Two endocardial heart tubes → 18th day.
3. Descends ventral to thorax region → 22–24th days.
4. Fusions of heart tubes → 22–24th days.
5. Cardiac looping → 24–28th days.
6. Wall of heart tube → 24–28th days.

Changes in Interior of the Heart

FATE AND DEVELOPMENT OF SINUS VENOSUS: MIDDLE OF 4–8TH WEEKS OF IUL

The formation of bulboventricular loop, i.e. cardiac loop C and then S shape is on 24–28th days. Sinus venosus initially caudal to primitive atrium, after cardiac looping, comes to lies dorsolateral to primitive atrium. Sinus venosus (4th week) consists of transverse portion via right and left horns. It maintains its paired condition. Middle of 4th week of IUL sinus venosus receives venous blood from entire embryo via right and left sinus horns.

Each horn receives 3 pairs of important veins

1. Vitelline or omphalomesenteric veins from yolk sac.
2. Umbilical veins carry oxygenated blood from placenta (lateral to vitelline veins).
3. Common cardinal veins (duct of Cuvier) from the cephalic (ACV) and caudal (PCV) parts of body wall.

Ventrally, sinus venosus communicates with primitive atrium through sinuatrial orifice. At first, communication between sinus venosus and primitive atrium is → sinuatrial orifice wide and central. Soon sinuatrial orifice entrance shifted to the right of primitive atrium.

Shift caused primarily by left to right shunt of blood which occurs in venous system during 5 weeks of IUL. Entire volume of blood conveyed by sinus venosus now reaches right half of primitive atrium via sinuatrial orifice.

1. Complete obliteration of right umbilical vein.
2. Obliteration of terminal part of left vitelline vein and left umbilical vein due to development of hepatic bud.
3. Left horn SV rapidly loses its importance.
4. Left common cardinal vein is obliterated by 10th week.
5. All that remains on the left sinus horn is coronary sinus and oblique vein of the left atrium.
6. Right horn → well developed.

To start initially 6 veins open in the sinus venosus: Tremendous alterations of the veins affect the interior of sinus venosus

1. Left to right shunt.
2. Appearance of hepatic bud in septum transversum.

   Supra-hepatic parts of left umbilical vein and left vitelline vein disappear.
3. Right umbilical vein degenerates completely.
4. Supra-hepatic parts of right vitelline vein form terminal part of inferior vena cava.
5. Presence of sub-hepatic LUV from placenta enters developing liver.
6. Presence of sub-hepatic vitelline veins from yolk sac enters developing liver later forms portal vein.

   Right horn and body of SV later incorporated into right atrium to form smooth posterior wall of right atrium.

Adult Veins

- Left common cardinal vein → oblique vein of the left atrium.
- Left horn of sinus venosus → coronary sinus.
- Right horn of sinus venosus enlarges and incorporated from smooth posterior part of right atrium.
- Terminal part right vitelline vein → final segment of IVC.
- Right common cardinal vein → SVC.

Entrance of sinuatrial orifice is flanked on each side by valvular fold → right and left venous valves

Dorsocranially these valves fuse forming the septum spurium:

1. Left venous valve and septum spurium fuse with developing atrial septum.
2. Superior portion of right venous valve forms crista terminalis.
3. Inferior portion of right venous valve forms valve for IVC and coronary sinus.

Crista terminalis forms dividing line between

1. Trabeculated anterior part of right atrium (primitive atrium)
2. Smooth posterior part of right atrium (sinus venarum which originates from right horn of sinus venosus).

   Four pulmonary veins from developing lung open into left part of primitive atrium.

Synopsis of Development and Fate of Sinus Venosus

1. Right horn and body of sinus venosus (sinus venarum) → posterior smooth part of right atrium.
2. Left horn and body of sinus venosus → coronary sinus.
3. Right duct of Cuvier → superior vena cava (lower part).
4. Left duct of Cuvier → oblique vein of Marshall
5. Supra-hepatic part of right vitelline vein→ terminal part of IVC.

20

Septum Formation in Common Atrium

Circulation before septation unidirectional → enters through venous end and leaves through arterial end. 18th, 24 to 28th days → corresponds to fusion of two endocardial heart tubes followed by cardiac looping within pericardial cavity.

Partitioning of Heart Begins at 5th Week and Ends by 8th Week

1. AV canal
2. Primordial atrium
3. Primordial ventricle

Major septa of heart are formed between 27 and 37th days (4–5th weeks of IUL). Septation of heart occurs simultaneously in all the chambers.

Separation occur between two atria, between two ventricles and between atria and ventricles.

The major septae are formed between 27 and 37th days of development. It is a simultaneous process

1. Septum formation in the AV canal
2. Septum formation in the common atrium
3. Septum formation in the truncus arteriosus and conus cordis
4. Septum formation in the common ventricle.

Endocardial Cushion

Endocardial cushions are contributed by migration of neural crest cells.

Neural crest cells are

1. Responsible for head and neck development (cartilage, bone and mesoderm of pharyngeal arches).
2. Contribute for endocardial cushions develop in atrio-ventricular and conotruncal regions.

   Teratogenic agents during this period (4–5th weeks) produce both craniofacial and cardiac defects.

In these locations assist in formation of

1. Atrial and ventricular septa (membranous portion).
2. Right and left AV canals and valves.
3. Aortic and pulmonary channels and valves.

I. **Partitioning of atrioventricular canal:** Towards the end of the 4th week (27th day). Endocardial cushions form on the dorsal and ventral walls of the AV canal. AV endocardial cushions approach each other and fuse, dividing the AV canal into right and left canals. These canals partially separate the primitive atrium from the ventricle.

II. **Partitioning of primordial atrium:** Beginning at the end of the 4th week (27th day). It is divided into right and left atria by the formation and fusion of two septa: Septum primum and septum secundum.

Summary of Intra-atrial Septum

Intra-atrial septum (IAS) develops from 3 sources:

1. Septum primum
2. Septum intermedium.
3. Septum secundum.

Right surface of IAS at birth presents

A. Fossa ovalis → septum primum.
B. Limbus fossa ovalis → septum secundum.

Left surface of IAS

A. Semilunar fold with concave upward septum primum.

B. Lunate depression → septum secundum.

Right atrium develops from 6 sources

1. Smooth posterior part (sinus venarum) behind crista terminalis develops from absorption of right horn of sinus venosus.
2. Upper part of right venous valve forms crista terminalis (demarcation).
3. Lower part of right venous valve forms valve of IVC and coronary sinus.
4. Anterior trabeculated rough part and auricle (atrial appendage) develop from right half of primitive atrium.
5. Inferior smooth part from right half of AV canal.
6. Intra-atrial septum from septum primum and septum secundum.

Left atrium develops from 4 sources

1. Smooth posterior part by absorption of pulmonary veins.
2. Anterior trabeculated rough part and auricle (atrial appendage) develops from left half of primitive atrium.
3. Inferior smooth part from left half of AV canal.
4. Intra-atrial septum from septum primum and septum secundum.

21

Primitive Ventricle and Bulbus Cordis

1. Development of membranous interventricular septum
   A. Endocardial cushions develop in atrioventricular canal (septum intermedium).
   B. Endocardial cushions in conotruncal regions.
2. Development of muscular interventricular septum.

AV–endocardial cushions fuse to form septum intermedium (5th week). The septum intermedium and minor lateral cushions divide the AV canal into right AV and left AV orifices. Completing dividing the AV canal into right and left orifices occur by 5th week. These canals partially separate the primitive atrium from the ventricle.

Simultaneously septum formation occurs in truncus arteriosus and conus cordis—5th week (truncal ridges). While growing both truncus ridges twist around each other and fuse and form a spiral septum → aortic pulmonary septum.

Aortic pulmonary septum twisting causes:

Proximally, pulmonary trunk lies anterior and ascending aorta lies posterior.

Distally, pulmonary trunk lies posterior and ascending aorta lies anterior.

Fused conus swellings and truncus septum together divides conus cordis

1. Anterolateral portion, outflow tract of right ventricle (smooth part of right ventricle).

2. Posteromedial portion, outflow tract of left ventricle (smooth part of left ventricle).

Primitive ventricle chamber forms rough part of left ventricle. Bulbus cordis chamber forms the rough part of right ventricle.

Septum Formation of Ventricles

1. Muscular part of the interventricular septum derives from the bulboventricular flange which is developed due to differential growth of primitive ventricle and bulbus cordis.

2. Membranous part of neural crest origin

   i. Connects upper free margin of the bulboventricular muscular IVS.

   ii. Derived from endocardial cushions of AV valve

   iii. Gets attached to lower border of spiral septum or the aorticopulmonary septum.

While septation in atrium is in progress, primitive ventricle also begins to expand.

This is accomplished by continuous growth of

A. Myocardium on the outside

B. Trabeculae formation inside.

Space between free rim of interventricular muscular septum and septum intermedium permits communication between two ventricles. Space is interventricular foramen.

Synopsis of Development of IVS 5–8th Weeks

Interventricular Septum Formed by 2 Sources

1. Muscular interventricular septum (floor of primitive ventricle).

2. Membranous part of interventricular septum

   i. Conus septum (formed by fusion of right and left bulbar ridges) forms upper part of intramembranous septum.

ii. Septum intermedium: Ventral (I) AV endocardial cushion forms lower part of intramembranous septum. Intramembranous septum derived from neural crest cells.

Development of Right Ventricle

A. Inflowing rough part formed by incorporated proximal part of bulbus cordis.
B. Outflow smooth dextroventral part of conus cordis (middle third of bulbus cordis).
C. IVS muscular and membranous parts.

Development of Left Ventricle

A. Inflowing rough part from left part of primitive ventricle.
B. Outflow smooth levodorsal part of conus cordis (middle third of bulbus cordis).
C. IVS muscular and membranous parts.

22

Development of Vascular System: Arterial System

Intraembryonic arteries and veins are first arranged in pairs (bilateral symmetrical).

Main alteration occurs

1. Fusion of paired vessels.
2. Hypertrophy of one vessel and atrophy of its counterpart.
3. New sprouts of vessels.

Arterial System

It consists of pair of dorsal aortae and 6 pairs of aortic arches, a pair of vitelline and umbilical arteries.

Aortic arches or brachial arch arteries are 6 pairs:

Aortic sac (ventral aorta) bifurcates into left and right horns. The 6 aortic arches arise from the aortic sac is distal part of truncus arteriosus pass through to pharyngeal arches (4–5 weeks). Terminate in the left and right dorsal aorta. Aortic arch arteries and pharyngeal arches appear in a cranial to caudal sequence. Primitive aorta (dorsal) intervene between notochord and dorsal wall of yolk sac.

Later two dorsal aortae with the head fold are connected to two horns of ventral aorta.

By 6 pairs of aortic arches. Two horns (limbs) of ventral aorta or aortic sac fuse caudally to form the truncus arteriosus which continuous with bulbus cordis. Cranial to developing heart, dorsal aorta remains paired where it is connected to ventral aorta, but caudal to this region these fuse to form single vessel. Initially each limb of ventral aorta is connected with dorsal aorta via 1st aortic arch.

With additional formation of branchial arches (4–5th weeks), additional aortic arches are formed.

Six pairs of aortic arches embrace the lateral wall of pharynx from ventral to dorsal aorta.

5th aortic arch pair either never forms, or forms incompletely and later regresses. Consequently 5 aortic arches are numbered I, II, III, IV and VI.

Caudally, two dorsal aortae fuse caudocranial to form single descending aorta from 4th lumbar segment to 4th thoracic segment form:

1. Thoracic aorta (T4–T12)
2. Abdominal aorta (T12–L4)
3. Median sacral artery (opposite 1st sacral segment).

Caudal to dorsal aorta bifurcates and continuous with umbilical arteries which carry deoxygenated blood from the embryo to placenta.

Fate of Aortic Arches

1. Aortic sac (ventral aorta) divides right and left horns and subsequently gives rise to right horn that forms brachiocephalic trunk. Left horn → proximal part of arch of aorta (between brachial carotid artery and left common carotid artery)
2. 1st aortic arch most of it disappears, but small part persists as maxillary artery (1st part).
3. 2nd aortic arch also disappears, but small part persists as stapedial and hyoid arteries.
4. 3rd aortic arch forms common carotid artery and first part of ICA. Remaining cranial part of ICA formed by cranial part of dorsal aorta. ECA is a sprout of 3rd aortic arch.
5. 4th aortic arch persists on both sides, ultimate fate is different on right and left side. Left side IV aortic arch forms arch of aorta between left common carotid artery (LCCA) and left subclavian artery (LSA).

6. Right side IV AA forms proximal segment of right subclavian artery and distal part formed by part of right dorsal aorta and right 7th intersegmental artery. Left subclavian artery → left 7th intersegmental artery. Upper limb bud is maintained by 7th intersegmental artery.

7. 5th aortic arch never forms.

8. 6th aortic arch is known as pulmonary arch gives off important branches to developing lung bud.

Right side → ventral part or right pulmonary artery. Distal part → loses its connection with dorsal aorta and disappears.

Left side → ventral part of left pulmonary artery. Dorsal part → persists during IUL as ductus arteriosus (ligamentum arteriosus).

Development of arch of aorta: 3 sources

1. Brachiocephalic trunk to LCCA → left limb of aortic sac.
2. LCCA to left subclavian artery → left 4th aortic arch.
3. left subclavian artery to origin of ductus arteriosus → left dorsal aorta.

23

Development of Venous System (4–8 Weeks)

Formation of SVC

Three major venous circuits like the arteries develop in a cephalocaudal direction are vitelline, umbilical and cardinal veins. With the development of the liver and mesonephric kidney profound affects in redirecting blood flow. Most of the venous blood is channeled from the left side to the right side of the body through the anatomizing vessels.

Cardinal venous complexes are somatic veins drain body wall consist of

A pair of anterior (pre) cardinal veins (ACVs) and a pair of posterior (post) cardinal veins (PCVs) which drain the rostral and caudal regions of embryo. ACV and PCV join to form short common cardinal vein (duct of Cuvier) that enters sinus venosus.

Formation of vena cava system (SVC and IVC) is characterized by appearance of anastomose between left and right veins

1. *Fate of sinus venosus:* Right horn of SV is incorporated into right atrium and left horn of SV forms coronary sinus.
2. Right common cardinal vein (RCCV) forms lower part of SVC. Left common cardinal vein forms oblique vein of left atrium.
3. *Superior vena cava formed:* RCCV: Lower part of SVC (intrapericardial part). Right anterior cardinal vein

(RACV) below the oblique anastomosis forms upper part of SVC.

4. *Fate of right anterior cardinal vein*
   - Cervical part (cranial to 7th intersegmental vein) becomes the right internal jugular vein.
   - Middle part gives rise to the right brachiocephalic vein.
   - Caudal part of RACV and RCCV forms the SVC.
   - Cranial part of RACV forms primary head veins which drain brain via → ACV, MCV and PCV and DV sinuses.

5. *Fate of left anterior cardinal vein*
   - Cervical part of LACV → internal jugular vein.
   - Cranial part of LACV → primary head veins (ACV, MCV and PCV).
   - Oblique anastomosis between two ACVs forms left brachiocephalic vein.

6. *Left side caudal LACV below the oblique channel*
   1. Left ACV forms left superior intercostal vein and ligament of left vena cava.
   2. Left CCV forms oblique vein of Marshall.
   3. Left horn sinus venosus forms coronary sinus.

24
Development of Venous System: Fate of Vitelline and Umbilical Veins

Formation of portal vein derived from vitelline veins and it drains GIT below diaphragm.

Vitelline veins follow the vitellointestinal duct, pass through septum transversum and drain into sinus venosus. Right and left vitelline veins arise from capillary plexuses of splanchnic mesoderm around yolk sac.

Vitelline veins traverse cranially on each of primitive duodenum, pass through septum transversum and end SV.

Hepatic cords appear and grow into septum transversum and interrupt the course of veins.

An extensive vascular network hepatic sinusoids are formed *in situ* which get connected to vitelline veins.

Portal vein (5–8 weeks) is formed by vitelline veins.

Vitelline veins are subdivided by hepatic bud in septum transversum into 3 parts: Infrahepatic, intrahepatic and suprahepatic.

Around U-shaped primitive duodenum loop, right and left vitelline veins are connected by 3 transverse anastomoses between right and left vitelline veins (form portal vein) in relation to primitive duodenum, the cephalic ventral, middle dorsal and caudal ventral anastomoses.

Primitive duodenum is encircled by figure of 8 anastomosis of vitelline veins.

When stomach rotates to right and duodenum also rotates to right.

Part of right vitelline vein between middle dorsal and cephalic ventral and middle dorsal anastomosis forms trunk of portal vein.

Splenic vein joins left end middle dorsal anastomosis. Superior mesenteric vein which drains primary intestinal loop derived from right vitelline vein joins splenic vein.

Fate of Vitelline Veins

1. Pre-hepatic part (infra) forms anastomosis around the duodenum which later on gives rise to the portal vein.

2. Hepatic part (intra) interrupted by the liver cords, forms tributaries of portal vein and hepatic vein → joins an extensive vascular network of hepatic sinusoids.

3. Post-hepatic part (supra): Upper part of LVV vein disappears.

   Subdiaphragmatic: Right and left veins form hepatic veins.

4. RVV (hepatic segment) → IVC.

Development of IVC, GIT, Respiratory, Urinary and Genital Systems

IVC is in adult composite vessel. Posterior cardinal veins are pair of longitudinal vessels along with dorsolateral aspect of mesonephric ridge.

Posterior cardinal veins, caudally receive iliac veins and cranially join common cardinal veins.

Major part of posterior cardinal veins, degenerates except cranial and caudal parts. The cranial part of right PCV: Arch of azygos that drains into SVC and caudal part of right PCV: Beginning of IVC. Caudal part of right PCV connected by transverse anastomosis with left PCV → left common iliac vein.

Gradually, the regression of posterior cardinal veins is replaced by two pairs of new longitudinal veins: Subcardinal and supracardinal veins.

1. A pair of subcardinal veins: Ventromedial to mesonephric ridge → drain the kidneys.
2. A pair of supracardinal veins lateral to sympathetic trunk → drain the body wall via intercostal veins (take over the function of PCV).

Subcardinal veins are connected

1. with each other by the subcardinal anastomosis,
2. with PCV through the mesonephros, and
3. with supracardinal veins through subcardinal–supracardinal anastomoses.

Right subcardinal vein from its cephalic end forms new channel dorsal to liver bud → hepatic cardinal channel → hepatic segment of IVC.

- Cranial part of right subcardinal vein → pre-renal segment of IVC.
- Left subcardinal vein regresses below renal veins.

Adult derivatives subcardinal veins forms:

- Stem of the left and right renal veins, suprarenal veins and gonadal veins.
- Two supracardinal veins connected with PCV cranially and caudally.
- Transverse anastomosis between subcardinal vein forms left renal vein.

Development of Inferior Vena Cava

Series of changes in the primordial veins

- Suprahepatic segment derived the right vitelline vein.
- Hepatic segment: Hepatorenal channel.
- Pre-renal segment: Right subcardinal vein
- Renal segment: Subcardinal and supracardinal anastomoses.
- Post-renal segment: Right supracardinal vein.
- Terminal segment: Right posterior cardinal vein.

DEVELOPMENT OF GIT: ENDODERM OF DEFINITIVE YOLK SAC

Cephalocaudal and lateral foldings of embryo, yolk sac is incorporated into the embryo to form the primitive gut tube. Two portions which remain outside the embryo are part of yolk sac and allantois. Primitive tubular gut extends from in median plane from buccopharyngeal membrane at the cephalic end to cloacal membrane at caudal end.

Primitive Gut and its Derivatives Discussed in 4 Parts

Pharyngeal gut → oropharyngeal membrane to respiratory diverticulum and it is part of foregut (head and neck).

Foregut → caudal to pharyngeal tube to the liver outgrowth.

Midgut → liver bud to junction of right two-thirds and left one-third of transverse colon in adult.

Hindgut → left one-third of transverse colon in adult to cloacal membrane.

Foregut

Endodermal gut tube of the yolk sac in head fold. Cranially foregut separated from stomadeum (primitive mouth cavity) by bilaminar buccopharyngeal membrane (14th day). Buccopharyngeal membrane (14th day) ruptures about 4th week and foregut communicates to exterior to stomadeum (primitive mouth cavity).

Caudally, foregut communicates with midgut via anterior intestinal portal (termination of bile duct II duodenum or liver bud).

Ventrally at pharyngeal esophageal junction foregut presents median laryngotracheal groove which leads to respiratory diverticulum (lung bud).

Foregut divided cephalic part (pre-laryngeal) → pharynx and definitive mouth and pharyngeal pouches (lateral wall).

Caudal part (post-laryngeal) → esophagus, stomach and duodenum I and II parts.

Midgut (Lateral Folds)

It extends from anterior to posterior intestinal portal (transverse colon or right two-thirds with left one-third → joins hindgut.

Midgut communicates with extraembryonic yolk sac by vitellointestinal duct.

Caecal diverticulum develops from midgut divides it pre-caecal segments (distal part of duodenum, jejunum and ileum) and post-caecal segments (caecum, appendix, ascending colon and transverse colon of right two-thirds).

Primary intestinal loop or midgut loop is the apex VI duct. It is also divided into superior mesenteric artery into pre-arterial (duodenum II, III and IV, J and most of I) and post-arterial segments (terminal I, C and A, AC and TC (right two-thirds).

Hindgut is Yolk Sac in Tail Fold of Embryo

Separated from surface by bilaminar cloacal membrane (16th day) ruptures on 7–8th weeks → opens to exterior the proctodeum.

From the ventral wall of allantoic diverticulum extends into umbilical cord.

Allantoic diverticulum divides hindgut into pre-allantoic part (distal part of transverse colon, descending colon and sigmoid colon) and post-allantoic part → dilates to form endodermal cloaca.

Endodermal Cloaca

Divided by urorectal septum into:
1. Dorsal part (primitive rectum)
2. Ventral part (primitive urogenital sinus)

Endodermal cloaca (post-allantoic part of hindgut)

1. Posterior part forms the rectum and upper part of anal canal.
2. Anterior part is primitive urogenital sinus forms mucous membrane of urinary bladder and urethra and part of vagina.

   Endodermal cloaca closed by cloacal membrane ruptures (7–8th weeks) and establishes GIT and urogenital system to exterior → proctodeum.

Primitive Gut

It is invested by splanchnopleuric layer of lateral plate of mesoderm of intraembryonic mesoderm.
1. Endoderm lining of yolk sac forms epithelium of the GIT, secretory and ductal cells of various glands, which secrete in the lumen including pancreas and liver.

2. Surrounding splanchnopleuric mesoderm forms the connective tissues, smooth muscles, blood vessels, lymphatics of the wall. Its external surface forms visceral peritoneum (absent in neck, thorax and hindgut as it traverses pelvic floor).
3. Associated neural elements invade the gut from neighboring neural crest cells.
4. Cranially, skeletal muscles are brachial arch origin (pharynx and esophagus, upper one-third).
5. Caudally, origin of musculature of the gut is uncertain (anal canal).
6. Structure of oral cavity and pharynx are partly muscular and partly bony.

Derivatives of Foregut

Below the diaphragm is supplied by celiac trunk:
1. Mucous membrane of tongue.
2. Epithelial lining of pharynx, esopharynx, stomach, duodenum up to ampulla of Vater.
3. Epithelial lining of respiratory system.
4. Auditory tube and tympanic cavity.
5. Parenchyma of tonsil, thyroid, parathyroid, thymus,
6. Liver and pancreas.

Derivatives of Midgut are Supplied by SMA

1. Epithelial lining of duodenum distal to ampulla of Vater, rest of small intestine, caecum, appendix, ascending colon and right two-thirds of transverse colon.
2. Meckel's diverticulum persists vitellointestinal duct.

Derivatives of Hindgut are Supplied by IMA

1. Mucous membrane of transverse colon from left one-third to upper part of anal canal (posterior part).
2a. Anterior part: Mucous membrane of urinary bladder, urethra and parenchyma of prostate (male)
2b. Epithelium of vagina (female).
3. Primitive sex cells derived from dorsal wall of hindgut.

Development of liver, gallbladder, ducts and pancreas—4th week liver, biliary apparatus (gallbladder and duct system), and pancreas are derived caudal part of endoderm of foregut.

Development of Liver

1. Parenchyma of liver: Endodermal hepatic bud arises from ventral wall to terminal wall of foregut (hepatocytes and intra-hepatic biliary duct system).
2. Fibrous stroma: Hematopoietic tissue and Kupffer cells, capsule and visceral peritoneum→ mesoderm of septum transversum.
3. Blood capillaries from vitelline to umbilical veins.

Development of the Pancreas (6–8th Weeks)

Pancreas begins to appear as two buds, dorsal pancreatic bud (26th day) and ventral pancreatic bud (28th day) from the endoderm of caudal part of foregut.

1. Dorsal bud develops from the dorsal wall of primitive duodenum, cephalic to hepatic bud and ventral bud extends dorsally and cranially in mesoduodenum and dorsal mesogastrium. It forms entire pancreas except lower part of head of pancreas.
2. Ventral bud develops from the hepatic bud at junction of foregut and midgut. Ventral bud is bilobed initially and later fuse into single mass forms lower part of head and uncinate process of pancreas.
3. Duct of ventral bud and distal part of the duct of the dorsal bud form the main pancreatic duct (Wirsung) that opens on the major duodenal papilla. Proximal part of the duct of the dorsal bud often persists as the accessory pancreatic duct (Santorini) that opens separately on the minor duodenal papilla.

DEVELOPMENT OF RESPIRATORY SYSTEM: 4TH WEEK OF IUL

Respiratory system has upper and lower parts. Upper respiratory system, i.e. nasal cavity and pharynx develops with development of face, oral cavity and pharyngeal arches. Lower respiratory system develops from lung bud → develops from foregut caudal to hypobranchial eminence.

Respiratory diverticulum (lung bud) appears 4th week of IUL. It develops from cranial part of foregut (yolk sac). Lung bud communicates with foregut via laryngotracheal orifice. Epithelium of internal lining of larynx, trachea, bronchi and lungs are entirely endodermal (i.e. foregut).

Cartilages, muscular and connective tissue of trachea and lungs are derived from splanchnic mesoderm. But larynx it derived from 4 to 6th pharyngeal arches.

Larynx develops from the cephalic part of laryngotracheal tube and communicates with pharynx. Internal lining of larynx originates endoderm of foregut. Laryngeal orifice changes from sagittal slit to a T-shaped opening. Cartilages and muscles of larynx develop mainly from mesoderm of 4th and 6th pharyngeal arches. All laryngeal muscles are innervated by branches of 10th cranial nerve (vagus nerve). Superior laryngeal nerve→ 4th pharyngeal arch (PA) and recurrent laryngeal nerve → 6th PA.

Trachea develops from intermediate part of laryngotracheal tube. Internal lining of trachea originates endoderm of foregut. Trachea cartilaginous rings and muscles → splanchnic pleuric mesoderm.

Lung develops from caudal part of lung bud. Lining epithelium derived from the endoderm (foregut). Cartilages, muscles and connective tissue develop mainly from splanchnopleuric mesoderm of pleuric cavity (intra-embryonic coelom). During separation of lung buds from the foregut forms trachea and two lateral outpockings → bronchial buds.

- At 4–5th weeks each bud enlarges to form right and left main bronchi.
- Right forms → 3 secondary bronchi (3 lobes)
- Left forms → 2 secondary bronchi (2 lobes)

Maturation of Lungs—6 Stages

1. Embryonic 4–8 weeks (2nd month): Development of trachea and major bronchi
2. Pseudoglandular 8–16 weeks (4th month): Development of remaining conducting airways (tertiary bronchi to terminal bronchiole).
3. Canalicular 16–28 weeks (7th month): Development of vascular bed and respiratory bronchiole.
4. Saccular 28–36 weeks (8th month): Formation of saccules.
5. Alveolar 36–40 weeks (term): Development of alveoli → to sustain gas exchange.
6. Post-term >41 weeks.

At birth, there are roughly 300 million alveoli. Between alveoli lie the parenchyma, composed of a double-layer of capillaries, that forms the primary septa. Before birth, lungs are filled with fluid, protein, mucus and surfactant which form phospholipid coat on alveolar membrane. At beginning of respiration (after birth), lung fluid is reabsorbed except surfactant coat which prevents alveoli collapsing during expiration.

DEVELOPMENT OF URINARY SYSTEM

Urogenital systems have a common development. Both develop from intermediate cell mass (mesoderm) and UGS (endoderm). Kidneys and ureters develop from (IM) and urinary bladder and urethra develop from UGS. Functionally urogenital system can be divided into 2 entirely different components: Urinary and genital systems. Embryologically and anatomically they are intimately interwoven with each other. Urinary system develops earlier.

Two systems develop from common mesodermal ridge → urogenital ridge (intermediate mesoderm), which develops on along the posterior abdominal wall.

Intermediate mesoderm extends craniocaudally on each side of dorsal aorta.

From cervical region to sacral region and project into dorsal wall of coelomic cavity.

It loses its connection with paraxial mesoderm.

Development of Kidneys and Ureters

Kidneys develop from 3 different overlapping systems → in craniocaudally sequence in the intermediate mesoderm.

1. Pronephros → rudimentary and non-functional.
2. Mesonephros functions for short period in fetal period.
3. Metanephros → forms permanent kidney.

Pronephros → transitory develops early part of 4th week. In human embryo, pronephros kidney appears in cervical and upper thorax of intermediate mesoderm. Represents 7–10 segmented arranged horizontal pronephric tubules and with single excretory pronephric duct. Pronephric duct grows caudally along nephrogenic cord and bends ventrally in urorectal septum and opens in primitive urogenital sinus. Pronephric tubules form vestigial nephrotomes regress before caudal ones are formed. By end of 4th week of IUL pronephric system disappears.

Mesonephric kidney starts later part of 4th week: Mesonephric kidney associated with disappearance of pronephric tubules and cephalic part of pronephric duct. Mesonephros develops caudal to pronephros. Disappears by 4th month completely, before its degeneration forms the gonads and suprarenal glands. Mesonephric kidney (later part of 4th week) replaces pronephric kidney and utilizes pronephric duct now known as mesonephric duct opens into urogenital sinus. Mesonephric tubules 70–80 are derived from intermediate mesoderm from the lower thoracic and upper lumbar regions. Each mesonephric tubule opens into pronephric duct (laterally) which now called *mesonephric duct or wolffian duct*. By 5th week → degeneration of proximal mesonephric tubules. Their duct proceeds caudally. Mesonephric kidney eliminates waste directly from blood by filtration.

Male (important) forms: Caudal mesonephric tubules form efferent ductules of testes.

Mesonephric duct→ canal of epididymis, vas deferens, seminal vesicles and ejaculatory duct.

Female forms: Mesonephric tubules disappear, but a few persist as tubules of epoöphoron and paraoophoron in broad ligament. Mesonephric duct → degenerates, if persists it is duct of Gartner which runs along side of uterus and opens into vagina.

Both female and male form

A. Trigone of urinary bladder
B. Ureteric bud forms ureter, collecting of system of kidney.

Metanephric Kidney: In Reptiles, Birds and Mammals

Metanephric kidney has selective reabsorption of glomerular filtrate back to blood because of loops of Henle. Metanephros appears in lumbosacral of intermediate mesoderm and persists as permanent kidney.

Human kidney develops from two parts

1. Collecting part: Ureteric bud develops earlier.
2. Secretory part develops metanephric blastema.
   Collecting part is from ureteric bud. It is outgrowth from the dorsomedial side of the caudal part of mesonephric duct, before it opens into the cloaca. Ureteric bud grows cranially and penetrates the metanephric blastema (nephrogenic cord). Ureteric bud cranially dilates and forms renal pelvis. Stalk of ureteric bud gives rise to ureter. Its dilated cranial end forms pelvis of ureter. It forms part of mesonephric duct between ureteric bud and cloaca is common excretory duct.

Excretory system of the kidney formed by ureteric bud (derived from mesonephric duct) gives rise

- Ureter
- Renal pelvis

- Major calyces
- Minor calyces
- 1–3 million collecting tubules and papillary ducts.

Excretory (secretory) part develops from metanephric blastema (intermediate mesoderm) by inductive influence of ureteric bud. It forms Bowman's capsule, PCT, loop of Henle and DCT. At birth, kidneys are lobulated. During infancy lobulation disappears as a result of growth. Metanephric kidney initially lies in pelvic cavity, opposite sacral segments receives arterial supply from median sacral artery. Gradually kidney ascends to abdominal cavity, lumbar region.

DEVELOPMENT OF URINARY BLADDER AND URETHRA (UROGENITAL SINUS: 4–7 WEEKS)

Mucous Membrane of Urinary Bladder

A. Entire mucous membrane of urinary bladder except trigone develops from the endoderm of vesicourethral canal of urogenital sinus.

B. Apex of urinary bladder is derived from absorption of proximal part of allantoic diverticulum (endodermal).

C. Trigone of urinary bladder develops from incorporation of caudal part of mesonephric ducts (mesoderm).

D. Trigone lateral angles receive ureters and inferior angle starts urethra.

E. Musculature (smooth) detrusor and other connective stromata are splanchnopleuric mesoderm which surrounds cloaca.

F. Neural elements—neural crest cells.

Initially bladder is continuous with allantois and distal part of lumen of allantois is obliterated to form thick urachus or median umbilical ligament which connects apex of urinary bladder to umbilicus.

Development of Male Urethra

A. Upper part of prostatic: Above ejaculatory ducts at the level of seminal colliculus dorsal wall from the mesoderm by incorporation of caudal parts of two mesonephric ducts.

B. Ventral wall (upper half) of prostatic urethra develops from vesicourethral canal of urogenital sinus.

C. Below the ejaculatory ducts both ventral and dorsal walls develop from pelvic part of UGS.

D. Membranous part of urethra is derived from endoderm of pelvic part of UGS.

E. Spongy part (penile) of urethra: It is associated with development of external genital development. It is derived from phallic part of UGS caudally close by UG membrane.

F. Urethra in glans penis, i.e. ectodermal.

G. Connective tissue and smooth muscle are derived from splanchnopleuric mesoderm around cloaca.

H. Neural elements: Neural crest cells.

Development of Female Urethra

• Entire ventral wall of urethra is mostly formed from vesicourethral canal of UGS (endodermal cloaca).

• Absorption of mesonephric duct (dorsal wall).

• It corresponds to prostatic urethra above the seminal colliculus.

GENITAL SYSTEM

Sex differentiation is complex process which involves many genes on X and Y chromosomes including some autosomes.

Genital systems are

• Development of gonads: Ovaries or testes

• Genital ducts: Male (mesonephric ducts) or female (paramesonephric ducts).

- External genitalia: Male type or female type.

Key for sexual dimorphism is Y chromosome. Y chromosome has testis determination factor (TDF) gene called the sex determination region Y (SRY). SRY gene on the short arm-Yp11. SRY protein is TDF, influence male development of embryo and its absence female development of embryo. Presence or absence of this TDF has direct effect on gonadal differentiation.

Sexual differentiation is chromosomal sex → gonadal sex → phenotypic sex.

Sex of the embryo is determined at the time of fertilization. Fetal gonads do not acquire male or female morphologic characteristics not until 7th week of IUL. The gonadal ridge or medial mesonephric ridge known as urogenital ridge. Indifferent gonad consists of inner medulla and outer cortex and it is lined by coelomic epithelium.

Indifferent gonad has 3 types of cells

1. Germ cells → primitive sex cells (endoderm)
2. Supporting cells → derived from coelomic epithelium of gonadal ridge (mesodermal) → Sertoli cells of testes or granulosa cells of ovary.
3. Stromal cells (mesoderm) → interstitial cells of Leydig (testis) or theca cells of ovary → derived from gonadal ridge.

During 7 weeks the gonads (genital ridge) begin to form testes in males (PGCs-XY), 8 weeks they begin to form ovaries in females (PGCs-XX).

DEVELOPMENT OF TESTIS

1. Primitive sex cells→ endoderm of hindgut.
2. Genital ridge (intermediate mesoderm) → seminiferous tubules, rete testis, sustentacular cells of Sertoli, interstitial cells of Leydig, fibrous septa and intrinsic coverings of testis.
3. Mesonephric tubules → efferent ductules.

4. Male genital duct system → mesonephric duct (wolffian duct) → canal of epididymis, vas deferens, seminal vesicles and ejaculatory ducts.
5. Appendix of testis → cranial end of paramesonephric duct.
6. Appendix of epididymis → cranial end of mesonephric duct.

DEVELOPMENT OF DEFINITIVE OVARY

1. Primordial germ cells endoderm of hindgut.
2. Middle part of genital ridge and cortex of genital ridge (intermediate mesoderm) → ovary.
3. Cephalic part forms suspensory ligament of ovary. Caudal part is incorporated in gubernaculum ovary.
4. Genital ridge forms the stroma of the ovary (follicular cells and tunica interna and externa → estrogen)
5. Duct system → paramesonephric (müllerian) system → uterine tube, uterus and upper one-third of vagina.

DEVELOPMENT OF GENITAL DUCTS: 4 TO 6TH WEEKS OF IUL

Both male and female embryos have two pairs of genital ducts. Mesonephric (wolffian) ducts (4th week) and paramesonephric (müllerian) ducts (6th week).

In male, mesonephric (wolffian) ducts form the male genital system (4th week).

Paramesonephric (müllerian) ducts regress.

In female, paramesonephric (müllerian) ducts (6th week) form female genital system.

Mesonephric (wolffian) ducts regress.

Mesonephric duct is formed with development of kidney.

Paramesonephric duct arises as a longitudinal invagination of coelomic epithelium on AL surface of urogenital ridge. Cranially the paramesonephric duct opens into coelomic cavity by a funnel shape. Caudally, the paramesonephric duct, it first runs lateral to mesonephric duct, then it crosses ventrally and grows caudomedially UGS. Caudal tip of continued ducts projects into the posterior wall of definitive urogenital sinus as müllerian tubercle or eminence (sinus tubercle).

Mesonephric ducts also open into definitive urogenital sinus on each side of müllerian tubercle after the absorption of its distal part by developing urinary bladder to form trigone.

Development of genital duct system and external genitalia occurs under influence of hormones circulating in the male fetus (46 XY) during IUL.

Synopsis of uterus development is entirely mesoderm

- Endometrium:
  1. Cephalic part of uterovaginal canal produced by fusion of caudal vertical part of paramesonephric duct → body and cervix.
  2. Incorporation of segment of horizontal parts → paramesonephric duct forms fundus of uterus.
  3. Myometrium: Mesenchyme around paramesonephric duct.
  4. Perimetrium and broad ligament: Pelvic fold (mesoderm).

Synopsis of uterus tube development is entirely mesoderm

1. Uterine tube (epithelium): Cephalic vertical and inter-mediate horizontal part of paramesonephric duct.
2. Muscles: Mesenchyme around paramesonephric duct.

Vaginal Development

1. Fornices of vagina → caudal fused vertical part of paramesonephric duct.
2. Upper four-fifths above hymen → sinovaginal bulbs (pelvic part of UGS—endodermal).
4. Lower one-fifth below hymen → vestibule: Phallic part of UGS.
5. External vaginal orifice → ectodermal.
6. Muscles → mesenchyme around paramesonephric duct.

MALE GENITAL DUCT SYSTEM: MESONEPHRIC DUCT: 4 WEEKS

Mesonephric ducts lie lateral to mesonephric ridge. Before its termination into cloaca (UGS), ureteric bud grows from it. Each mesonephric duct (medial to paramesonephric duct) extends caudal wards from mesonephric tubules to dorsal wall of UGS through urorectal septum.

Craniomost end of mesonephric duct in male persists appendix of epididymis.

Mesonephric ducts in male persist craniocaudally as

- Canal (duct) of epididymis → body and tail.
- Ductus deferens (vas deferens) and seminal vesicle.
- Ejaculatory duct which opens into pelvic part of UGS.

Gonadal ridge (mesodermal): Primary sex cords derived from medulla → seminiferous tubules, rete testes, tunica albuginea, Leydig cells and Sertoli cells.

Primordial germ cells (endoderm of hindgut) form the spermatogonic series of cells.

Development of the male reproductive tract

- Under the influence of SRY, the gonad develops into a testis containing spermatogonia, Leydig cells, and Sertoli cells.
- Leydig cells produce testosterone, which supports growth of the mesonephric ducts.

  Note: Without testosterone, the mesonephric ducts will regress.

- Some testosterone is converted into dihydroxytestosterone (DHT), which supports development of the prostate gland, penis, and scrotum.
- Sertoli cells produce anti-müllerian hormone which induces regression of the paramesonephric ducts.

  Note: In the absence of MIS, the paramesonephric ducts will persist.

External Genitalia

- Genital folds
- Genital tubercle elongates from phallus
- Two pairs of mesodermal swellings lateral to genital folds are genital swellings and labioscrotal swellings.

External Genitalia in Male

At the indifferent stage, the SRY gene on the Y chromosome encodes for the expression of testis determining factor. The testes are formed and testosterone and MIS are released.

Stimulate the mesonephric ducts to form the male genital duct system.

Testosterone induces the formation of male external genitalia

1. Development of external genitalia in male is under the influence of androgens secreted by fetal testis which causes the rapid elongation of genital tubercle or phallus to penis.
2. 3rd month: Two genital folds (urethral folds) close beneath endodermal urethral cells and completes floor of penile part of urethra.
3. Genital swellings form scrotal swellings arise in inguinal region.

   Move caudally and each swelling make half of scrotum separated by scrotal septum.

External Genitalia in Female

Factors controlling the female external genitalia are very clear.

At the indifferent stage, there is no SRY gene, so the ovary forms.

No testosterone and no MIS: The paramesonephric ducts form female genital ducts. No testosterone but estrogen induces the formation of female external genitalia. However, esotrogen play an important role.

1. Genital tubercle elongates slightly to form clitoris.
2. Genital folds do not fuse and develop labia minora.
3. Genital swellings enlarge and do not fuse and develop labia majora. Urethral groove between urogenital membrane and genital folds form vestibule. Female urethra opens anteriorly below clitoris. Vagina opens posterior to urethra.